Praise for the South African edition of

The Journey to Pain Relief

—◦◊◦—

"This book is a valuable contribution to pain management and deserves to be promoted internationally."

— PROFESSOR DAVID NIV, President of the World Institute of Pain
Professor and Chairman, Centre for Pain Medicine
Sourasky Medical Centre, Tel Aviv, Israel

"In her introduction Phyllis Berger indicates that the book is dedicated to all patients with pain. It is very difficult for an author to write a medical book with appeal for both the patient with pain and health professionals involved in its management. However, she has done this admirably. She takes the reader into the gloomy caverns of pain and suffering, throwing light into the darkest of corners as she goes."

— CHARLES LIGGINS, Chairman of the Allied Health
Professions Council of South Africa
Editor of *Meridian,* the newsletter of the Acupuncture
Association of the South African Society of Physiotherapy

"A South Africa–based author, Phyllis Berger, has authored *The Journey to Pain Relief,* a book that will prove helpful to those who suffer from chronic pain. Indeed, the author, a physiotherapist and acupuncture expert herself, suffered from pain following a spinal fusion of the upper cervical vertebrae in 1992. Her book is a mix of mainstream and holistic approaches to pain treatment with chapters covering a variety of treatments. Whether it is headaches, advice on posture improvement, or recovering from various accidents, this is a thorough look at the subject of pain reduction and cure."

— one of BOOKVIEWS picks of the month, see www.bookviews.com

Dedication

———◦◦◦———

This book is dedicated to all patients with pain.

Ordering

Trade bookstores in the U.S. and Canada please contact:

> Publishers Group West
> 1700 Fourth Street, Berkeley CA 94710
> Phone: (800) 788-3123   Fax: (510) 528-3444

Hunter House books are available at bulk discounts for textbook course adoptions; to qualifying community, health-care, and government organizations; and for special promotions and fund-raising. For details please contact:

> Special Sales Department
> Hunter House Inc., PO Box 2914, Alameda CA 94501-0914
> Phone: (510) 865-5282   Fax: (510) 865-4295
> E-mail: ordering@hunterhouse.com

Individuals can order our books from most bookstores, by calling **(800) 266-5592**, or from our website at **www.hunterhouse.com**

THE JOURNEY TO PAIN RELIEF

A Hands-On Guide to Breakthroughs
in Pain Treatment

Phyllis Berger

Hunter House
PUBLISHERS

> Hunter House Inc., Publishers
> PO Box 2914
> Alameda CA 94501-0914

Library of Congress Cataloging-in-Publication Data

Berger, Phyllis, BSc.
    The journey to pain relief : a hands-on guide to breakthroughs in pain
treatment / Phyllis Berger. — 1st U.S. ed.
       p. cm.
    "First published in South Africa in 2003 as The Journey to Pain Relief."
    Includes bibliographical references.
    ISBN-13: 978-0-89793-469-5
    ISBN-10: 0-89793-469-5
    1. Pain—Alternative treatment—Popular works. 2. Acupuncture.
3. Self-help techniques. I. Title.
RB127.B469 2006   2006020291
616'.0472—dc22

Project Credits

Cover Design: Peri Poloni-Gabriel,
  Knockout Books
Book Production: Jinni Fontana
Developmental and Copy Editor: Gordon Kelley
Copy Editor: Kelley Blewster
Proofreader: John David Marion
Indexer: Nancy D. Peterson
Acquisitions Editor: Jeanne Brondino

Editor: Alexandra Mummery
Senior Marketing Associate: Reina Santana
Rights Coordinator: Candace Groskreutz
Customer Service Manager: Christina Sverdrup
Order Fulfillment: Washul Lakdhon
Administrator: Theresa Nelson
Computer Support: Peter Eichelberger
Publisher: Kiran S. Rana

Printed in Canada by Transcontinental Printing

9 8 7 6 5 4 3 2 1   First U.S. Edition   07 08 09 10 11

CONTENTS

Contents

Contents

Contents

Important Note

The material in this book is intended to provide a review of resources and information related to chronic pain. Every effort has been made to provide accurate and dependable information. However, professionals in the field may have differing opinions, and change is always taking place. Any of the treatments described herein should be undertaken only under the guidance of a licensed health-care practitioner. The author, editors, and publishers cannot be held responsible for any error, omission, professional disagreement, outdated material, or adverse outcomes that derive from use of any of the treatments or information resources outlined in this book, either in a program of self-care or under the care of a licensed practitioner.

Foreword

Chronic-pain management, as espoused by the universally acknowledged father of pain medicine, the late John Bonica, M.D., is a multidisciplinary exercise that attempts to control pain in patients who have not responded to conventional medical modalities. Implementing comprehensive chronic-pain management can require assimilating many disciplines to achieve success. This can become bureaucratically unwieldy and may be financially impractical. As a result, some fragmentation of the principles espoused by Dr. Bonica more than forty years ago has occurred, and unidisciplinary "pain clinics" have become commonplace. For example, physical therapy was considered to be essential in the administration of an effective pain clinic; today physical therapy usually stands alone or is part of a rehabilitation program. Phyllis Berger has almost single-handedly highlighted the importance of physical therapy in contemporary chronic-pain management in South Africa, and she has done so in a scholarly, effective, and easy-to-implement manner. The field of chronic-pain management has been significantly enhanced by her work.

I have known Phyllis Berger for more than fifteen years. Her commitment to studying the basic sciences and clinical sciences relating to pain management, as well as her intellectual acuity, has made her unique among her peers. Her resolve to develop effective pain therapies began in South Africa when it was not trendy, rewarding, or fashionable to do so. Nevertheless, she persisted relentlessly in her dedication to her patients and in her acquisition of new knowledge to hone her skills as a practicing physical therapist with a special interest in pain management.

It was during her many travels to international conferences that I had the good fortune to meet with her and observe her scholarly intuitiveness regarding pain medicine. I am truly impressed with her knowledge and her understanding of the principles of medicine in general, and those of pain medicine in particular. She has demonstrated terrific organizational skills, not only through the building of her own clinic in Johannesburg, but also in her dedication to sharing her knowledge with her colleagues and, more importantly, her patients.

In the United States today, few pain clinics have physical therapy incorporated within their operational structure. Some of the reasons for that are purely economic, and one has to recall the draconian event, i.e., the Balanced Budget Act of 1997 (BBA 97), in which the reimbursements to health-care providers were significantly reduced in an attempt to balance the U.S. federal budget. As a result of these measures, most clinics could not afford a physical therapist within their structure, and the most ideal arrangement was to have a referral relationship with a particular physical therapist. The quality of care for chronic-pain patients has diminished as a result of this action.

I hope that *The Journey to Pain Relief* will enlighten both health-care providers and patients about the usefulness of physical therapy in the overall management of chronic pain. It is well demonstrated in this text that physical therapy can play a major role in the management of most musculoskeletal pain. The rehabilitative value of physical therapy in selective neurogenic pain is also emphasized. The maintenance of a healthy muscle unit and, by extension, a healthy nerve/muscle unit, acts as an important basis not only for controlling chronic musculoskeletal pain but also for preventing the development of acute and chronic pain syndromes.

Phyllis Berger has drawn from her broad experience in treating chronic-pain patients to outline various strategies and therapeutic techniques for the practical daily management of chronic pain. I am sure all readers will be impressed with the way she integrates pain management with various physiological functions while showing the connection between the failure of that function and various pathological states. The way she deals with issues like stress, fatigue, inflammation, the immune system, coping skills, and suffering attests to her thorough understanding and deep knowledge of pathophysiological and psychosocial factors that directly and indirectly affect chronic pain. In this text she offers simple but poignant hints on stretching exercises and effective therapeutic modalities from which therapists and patients alike can benefit.

This book helps both chronic-pain patients and physical therapists "connect the dots" and shows the practical relevance of alternative modalities in providing comprehensive pain management. The clarity, thoroughness, and depth of this work serve to break down perceived barriers to practicing comprehensive, multidisciplinary pain medicine. She effectively combines clinical issues with practical applications while focusing on the patient, the pain, and its impact on various socioeconomic and/or psychosocial factors that may ultimately affect the patient's pain and suffering. This concept is well illustrated in the many case histories used throughout the text.

Phyllis has explored acupuncture and electrical stimulation analgesia (ESA) with the scholarly approach that it requires, yet her discussions are so complete and detailed that these modalities are made "user-friendly" and easy to administer. Patients, as a consequence, may feel less intimidated and fretful about the scope and potential efficacy of these techniques.

I would like to congratulate Phyllis Berger on *The Journey to Pain Relief* and assure her of its potential to make a significant long-term contribution to the field of pain medicine. The benefit of her knowledge, as presented in this book, extends not only to providers but also to those ever-inquiring patients who in this computer-driven environment continue to explore the Internet and other sources for greater knowledge on the mechanisms and treatment of chronic-pain syndromes. I have no doubt that all readers will appreciate this text.

— WINSTON C.V. PARRIS, M.D., FACPM, CMG

Foreword to the South African Edition

With outstanding insight Phyllis Berger chose a travel metaphor for the title of this book on the multiple modalities of pain relief. Pain is at home; relief from pain is a distant port-of-call. Getting from here to there will take some effort.

If you have a body part that just won't stop hurting, or generalized aches and pains that limit your activity and sap the joy of living, you are not alone. Researchers consistently report that nearly 50 percent of adults have experienced recurrent or persistent pain, and nearly 20 percent say they experience significant chronic pain—pain that is bad enough to interfere with daily living. The most common pains are headaches and migraine; back, shoulder, and neck pain; aching joints; bellyaches and heartburn; and generalized dull pains that seem to be everywhere. As life expectancy increases, the number of individuals who endure chronic pain is expected to continue increasing. There's a good chance that you or someone you know has experienced persistent pain. Recurrent and persistent pain is so prevalent that many people regard it as unavoidable, as part of the normal wear and tear of being alive. This does not have to be the case.

Traditionally, physical pain has been a matter squarely within the medical realm. When it comes to acute, short-lasting pain, medicine has a variety of powerful and reliable remedies. For example, since the invention of anesthesia in the mid-nineteenth century, surgical operations are no longer the horror they once were. Everyday aches and bruises are effectively eased using over-the-counter pain relievers. And pain after trauma and surgery can be controlled by strong analgesics.

The problem is with chronic pain. Analgesic drugs have serious, sometimes life-threatening side effects when they are used for months or years at a stretch. There are second- and third-line medical therapies, such as anticonvulsant and antidepressant medicines and various invasive procedures, but these tend to have even more adverse side effects than the first-line drugs. Furthermore, they can be expensive, and far too often they just don't work well.

The pervasiveness of chronic pain despite dramatic advances in other domains of medicine has contributed to the tremendous growth in recent years of various paramedical and nonmedical healing arts. This growth is fostered by authors like Phyllis Berger who provide essential tools to the growing number of people with the gumption to do something about their pain when conventional medicine proves impotent. There is no sharp border between medicine and healing. And the dividing line continues to blur as major hospitals and health-care providers begin to offer modalities such as acupuncture and stress-reduction techniques.

In *The Journey to Pain Relief,* Phyllis Berger has done us all a service by collecting in one volume a remarkable variety of proposed treatment options. Her stated aim is to empower chronic-pain sufferers and those who care for them. Empowerment, she explains, comes from understanding what causes pain, comprehending its effects on body and soul, and gaining access to an armamentarium of modalities that may provide pain relief. Her book is unusual and praiseworthy within the large genre of books on healing for two reasons:

- First, her primary aim is to empower her readers rather than herself. This is not one of the hundreds of books out there trying to convince you that a particular treatment, machine, or diet is the best and therefore the one you should buy and use. Rather, this is an annotated collection of potentially helpful therapies. You choose.

- Second, she has gone out of her way to present evidence from the published literature backing up claims that particular techniques do indeed work. Phyllis Berger has the heart of a scientist, and she expresses respect for her readers by presenting the evidence, such as it is, in a digestible manner. It is important to her that the source of authority not be based in mysticism, charisma, celebrity status, or even academic certification. What carries weight for her is understanding, experimentation, and documentation.

Which brings us to the crux of the matter: Do these therapies actually help to relieve pain? The short answer is yes, but let me elaborate....

I am a scientist who specializes in the biological mechanisms of chronic pain. This is my training and this is my job. Believe me, science is difficult. It can be very hard to prove things authoritatively. This difficulty is greatly compounded when such proof concerns subjective feelings like pain.

In the days of the Bible, authority was established by performing miracles. Precisely because of the numerous "miracles" of modern science, we tend to attach an aura of authority to anyone who claims to be a scientist or who uses scientific results to bolster his or her claims. But unless the claim is as indisputable as a moon landing, it is often difficult for a nonscientist to evaluate the validity of scientific evidence. It isn't always easy for a scientist either. Errors of evaluation are frequently made, even by professional scientists.

Beyond the matter of false or exaggerated claims, the question of whether a particular therapy works depends to a considerable degree on what is meant by the word "works." It is perfectly reasonable to use as a criterion whether the particular "therapy" in question, be it the use of magnetic fields or prayer, is better at relieving pain than doing nothing. To her credit, Phyllis Berger maintains that it is essential to first establish that the pain is not due to a medically treatable cause such as a tumor or an infection. But after that has been done, empowering yourself by doing something active to try to improve your pain is far better than sitting around and moping. Initiative and a positive attitude can help, irrespective of whether the magnets have any physiological effect or whether anyone will hear your prayers.

Additionally, trying an "alternative" approach to pain relief is likely to have nonspecific pain-relieving effects. I am referring to the famous placebo effect. Remarkable as it may seem, it is a well-documented and increasingly well-understood fact that any action may relieve your pain if you anticipate that it could do so. Of essence is the belief in pain relief. It doesn't matter much why you believe. Belief, for example, may derive from something you were told, usually by someone whose authority you accept. Or it may derive from a prior good experience (conditioning), or from reading the results of a scientific experiment. Importantly, the placebo effect does not depend on whether the scientific results you read, or the information you were given, is true. What counts is your belief and your expectation.

The placebo effect is a blessing, not something you should see as primitive or undignified. For it to work best, it is important not only that the patient believe that the treatment in question has a good chance of working, but also that the therapist share this conviction. It is here in particular that Phyllis Berger has made a real contribution by bringing together a rich potpourri of putative pain-relieving techniques. Irrespective of biological actions, some of these work better with some therapists/healers than others, and with some patients than others. There are numerous reasons why a particular therapist, or a particular client, may be inclined to believe that magnets will work while prayer won't, for example, or that acupressure is more likely to be effective than circularly polarized laser radiation. The reason doesn't matter; the anticipation and belief do. With so many therapeutic modalities to choose from, there is bound to be at least one that resonates with you.

The placebo effect is a much maligned concept. Yet it is a fact that whenever powerful, proven pain relievers are given, a significant proportion of the analgesic effect obtained is due to the placebo effect. For example, people given morphine benefit from both a substantial pharmacological effect and a hefty placebo effect. In experiments in which subjects are convinced by (false) words or by a bogus demonstration that a drug will have little analgesic effect, the actual effect is greatly diminished, even if the drug happens to be as pharmacologically effective as morphine. Lack of belief can actually deprive you of a significant part of the pain relief offered by otherwise powerful painkillers.

There have been instances when well-established invasive procedures for pain relief, even surgery, turned out to have no analgesic effect beyond that of the placebo. Sadly, in a sense, these previously powerful pain-relieving procedures tend to lose their effect the minute therapist and patient no longer believe they are effective.[1]

In drug-efficacy trials the pharmacological effect of a drug is typically evaluated in a randomized placebo-controlled trial. Neither the patients nor the doctors know who received the drug and who received the placebo. It is almost always noted in such trials that placebo-treated patients obtain a measure of pain relief. This happens because whether a participant receives drug or placebo, there is a certain degree of expectation that relief might be obtained, and hence a certain amount of placebo effect.

In clinical trials run by drug companies, attempts are usually made to minimize expectations, and hence to minimize the placebo effect. Imagine what would happen if both the experimental and the placebo control groups were told they were to receive the real pain reliever: The placebo effect would strengthen in both groups, the pharmacological effect of the drug would remain the same, and hence the apparent benefit of the drug would appear to be reduced. This scenario can be pushed even further. Imagine that members of the placebo group are told they will receive a powerful analgesic drug, and those in the experimental group are told they will receive placebo. The placebo group could conceivably obtain more pain relief than the drug group! Placebo analgesia is a real biological effect, no less real or biological than the effects of pharmaceutical pain relievers.

What can be said about the biological effects of the healing modalities reviewed in *The Journey to Pain Relief* beyond their nonspecific motivating and placebo effects? There are two answers. The first is that very few of these pain-relief techniques, if any, have passed scrutiny in randomized placebo-controlled trials. As a result we lack data solid enough to satisfy scientists of the ilk who can send rockets to the moon. For better or for worse, few public or private resources are devoted to high-quality clinical trials of healing modalities. Rigorous tests of the efficacy of drugs, devices, and procedures are difficult and costly to perform, whether the modality to be tested is a conventional medical treatment or an alternative healing option.

The second answer routinely raises animosity among healers who are not skilled scientists. While rigorous trials may be necessary to definitively prove efficacy, they are not the only way to predict the likelihood that a proposed therapy will turn out to have efficacy beyond the nonspecific. Fairly good predictions of efficacy can also be made based on a theoretical understanding of the biological processes in question. Claims of bending spoons with the power of thought, for example, or of levitation through meditation are not impossible a priori. They simply require new physical principles. Since it is so rare an event that a new physical principle is actually established, scientists of the sort who are qualified to get a rocket to the moon are not inclined to take seriously the frequent claims of stage entertainers and New Age enthusiasts of phenomena that depend on new physical principles. This is the reason why they tend to be cool about investing resources in testing/debunking such claims. If even a single such claim were adequately documented, and a new physical principle thereby established, the skeptical attitude of hard scientists would change. This is the status of many, although not all, of the healing modalities discussed in *The Journey to Pain Relief.*

Wise practitioners of so-called "alternative medicine" are able to put aside affront and animosity and avoid getting sucked into debates with scientists on their turf. Although the modalities described by Phyllis Berger may not be scientifically proven or provable in randomized clinical trials, the fact is that they do help people, day in and day out, to obtain a measure of pain relief. They help individuals to take an active interest in their own welfare, and they work by the various biological and psychological effects associated with the belief that they *can* work. These are solid benefits, irrespective of the unresolved issue of additional biological or physical effects.

With the great variety of putative pain-relief modalities presented in *The Journey to Pain Relief,* on what basis should a prospective patient or therapist choose a particular technique? There are three keys:

1. Make a list of the modalities that you think are most likely to work. This may sound like an impossible mission, an invitation to train as a scientist and undertake proper clinical trials. But, in fact, what needs to be done is easy. Simply read *The Journey to Pain Relief,* and choose the modalities that appear most convincing to you on the basis of your own knowledge and beliefs, as well as of what you are able to learn from reading and talking to others. Remember that the expectation of success by both therapist and patient is important. It is hard to fake it; unspoken signals can pass from therapist to patient and undermine efficacy.[2] If you are a therapist and both you and your patient believe it will work, it probably will. Moreover, if you believe it, you can tell your prospective patient that it is likely to work without being dishonest.

2. From the list of healing modalities you have just made in step 1, eliminate the ones that carry the greatest potential risks. Avoid chemical agents that are ingested, including natural products, if they have not been fully tested for safety, invasive procedures for which your therapist has not been professionally trained, anything that uses high-power energy, and anything that causes significant pain.

3. Finally, depending on the financial means of patient and practitioner, eliminate from your list the modalities that are so expensive that they risk being exploitative. In the realm that we are discussing, expensive things do not necessarily work better than inexpensive ones. The possibility of exploitation in nonfinancial ways also needs to be considered.

As Phyllis Berger explains so well, the methods described in *The Journey to Pain Relief* empower both patient and therapist by putting a road map in their hands that is likely to lead them to pain relief. The journey is not necessarily easy, and it may involve some false starts. But it is well worth undertaking.

Keep at it, and don't lose hope.

— MARSHALL DEVOR, PH.D.
Professor, Institute of Life Sciences and Center for Research on Pain
Hebrew University of Jerusalem, Israel

References

1. Gracely, R.H. 2000. Charisma and the art of healing: Can nonspecific factors be enough?" In *Proceedings of the 9th World Congress on Pain: Progress in pain research and management* vol. 16, ed. M. Devor, M.C. Rowbotham, and Z. Wiesenfeld-Hallin, 1045–67. Seattle, WA: IASP Press, 2000.

2. Ibid.

PREFACE

My qualifications on the subject of pain come not only from my professional experience as a physiotherapist and an acupuncturist, but also from the fact that I myself have been a pain sufferer.

Observing and interacting with patients who are in pain moves and disturbs me. I become deeply distressed by their plight and by the suffering and desperation they often experience. Some of my patients have gone through many dreadful experiences. These include the condition itself as well as myriad investigations, procedures, and treatments, which often produce no change and can even worsen their condition.

As for myself, I experienced intolerable pain when I was inadequately medicated after a spinal fusion of the upper cervical vertebrae (C2 to C4) in 1992. At the time, I felt as if my whole body was exploding with severe, unbearable pain—I could not believe that a person could suffer such agony! Prior to my surgery, I had endured many years of neck pain and compressed nerves. Two years before I developed the problem in my neck that prevented me from comfortably doing mundane tasks or even holding my head upright— the same problem for which I underwent surgery—my eighteen-year-old daughter became critically ill. I have since discovered that many people experience sad and disturbing events within a couple of years before developing a severe illness, such as cancer, or other physical problems. When I first experienced my crises in family and health, medical science had not yet scientifically validated the link between emotional and physical disorders.

In the late nineties, I again entered a very difficult time. My personal life changed dramatically and I developed low-back pain that ultimately persisted for more than three years. This time, however, there was no way I was going the route of surgery, as I now understood the connection between my physical and emotional well-being. I opted for psychological therapy, aura healing, stretching (via tai chi classes), Pilates, walking on a treadmill, electrical stimulation, acupuncture, and the occasional anti-inflammatory medication.

Through my own experiences, as well as through implementing treatments I devised for others, I have discovered that there is hope and help for many pain sufferers. It is important to emphasize, however, that chronic-pain patients only achieve success when they are determined to help themselves, which involves making an effort to find out what helps, both physically and mentally. Their success becomes an example to others. Finally, a successful patient becomes a happy person…and a happy person becomes a healthy one!

Unfortunately, neither the average layperson nor the average medical professional has sufficient information on the range of therapies available to treat pain. I believe that informing therapists and medical professionals of the value of alternative options will ultimately provide patients with a wider spectrum of treatment possibilities. Toward this end, after many years of working in pain clinics and in a physiotherapy, acupuncture, and rehabilitation clinic, and after treating countless patients with different types of pain, I decided to analyze the treatments that had been successful and the methods I had used to manage my own pain. The result is *The Journey to Pain Relief*.

This book can be used by patients as a self-help guide. It provides information and explanations about chronic pain, about different types of treatments, and about various coping skills that will return a sense of control to their lives. It also provides useful information for medical professionals so they can more fully understand and more effectively treat their chronic-pain patients.

It aims to offer both a journey of self-discovery and a route to pain relief.

A Professional Journey

I would like to describe the path that led me to explore the field of pain management. I qualified in physiotherapy in 1966 at the University of the Witwatersrand, in Johannesburg, South Africa. I was interested in rehabilitation, and from my earliest experiences of treating patients, I wished that a set of exercises could be developed to help every condition. I had a suspicion that this could be the answer to many problems. Today, it is exciting to see that many exercise programs are widely available, such as hydrotherapy, water aerobics, training at health clubs, and Pilates classes. People are indulging in these various activities—and getting better!

My first position as a physiotherapist was in a private practice in Johannesburg. I had to resign after six months, however, due to the arrival of my first child. Five years later, I started my own small practice in my home, armed only with an ultrasound machine, an ice pack, and, of course, my two hands. It was a learning experience. I spent many years treating all kinds of conditions, from chest complaints to bad backs and sore knees. I also taught prenatal classes.

Two things frustrated me about physiotherapy. The first was that rehabilitation after injury or surgery was a lengthy process for many patients. I felt that if only I could go deeper, find other methods to improve strength, or reach the specific point of the problem, I could achieve more rapid results.

The other issue was that after many treatments involving extensive mobilization, massage, and even traction, patients sometimes continued to have headaches or back pain. I often ran into these patients in the supermarket or elsewhere, and some reported that they had improved *only* after they had started walking or exercising in the gym.

I designed classes to teach patients back exercises and other aspects of back care, which I called "Back School." I gave each patient a list of appropriate exercises to do at home. When I met these patients, even years later, they would often report that their backs were fine, as long as they did their exercises. Unfortunately, everyday demands tend to take over, leading to inconsistency and lagging commitments, and eventually most patients just stopped doing their exercises. When their backs became painful, they would follow their exercise program again, with positive results. I was certain that if patients enjoyed exercise, they would do it consistently and it would become a way of life instead of part of a treatment. A person should not "feel like a patient" but rather like a healthy person choosing a healthy lifestyle.

The next milestone in my professional life was my exposure to acupuncture. I attended my first acupuncture course at the Johannesburg General Hospital in 1989. I was fascinated by this ancient art of medicine and completed all the courses available to physiotherapists in South Africa. I spent another two years studying traditional Chinese medicine and obtained a South African diploma in acupuncture in 1995.

Acupuncture opened up new vistas of treatment to me and explained many of the problems I had encountered in treating patients through physiotherapy alone. It also helped me treat my patients more efficiently and more successfully. I found that a needle placed in a strategic position could produce profound effects on pain, movement, and the behavior of the individual. It was acupuncture that drew me into the arena of pain treatment.

During my acupuncture courses, I was also introduced to the concept of electricity as a healing modality. To my surprise, I discovered that certain direct currents and electrical stimulation of muscles, although painful for the patient, reduced the period of healing and rehabilitation. I also realized that not all currents helped every person or every condition, and that I would have to learn more about electric currents and magnetic fields and their effect on the human body. In particular, I discovered a device for the delivery of an electric current that seemed to rapidly relieve pain: the transcutaneous electrical nerve stimulation (TENS) unit.

In 1994, I was invited to join Professor Selma Braude (a radiologist specializing in radiation therapy for cancer) and Liz Human (a radiographer and organizer of the Cancer Radiation Department of the Rand Clinic, in Johannesburg) as a consultant in a multidisciplinary pain clinic. This was the first private pain clinic in Johannesburg. The staff included a psychologist. Later that same year I joined Professor Ted Shipton in founding the Rand Multidisciplinary Pain Clinic, which was part of the Rand Clinic hospital, in Hillbrow. Professor Shipton is an anesthetist and physician who also directed the Pain Relief and Research Unit at the University of the Witwatersrand.

During the years that I worked with Professor Shipton, we were both fascinated by the effects that electric currents, acupuncture, and rehabilitation had on chronically ill and desperately afflicted pain patients. Over the next few years I attended many conferences on pain and took courses on acupuncture in Latvia, Israel, the United Kingdom, Australia, Cyprus, Spain, and other countries. I also joined many societies involved in researching pain, such as the International Association for the Study of Pain and the World Institute of Pain Clinicians. In 1998, I was privileged to participate in research on modified direct current (MDC), a form of electric current that is produced by an apparatus called the action potential simulation current device (APS). It fascinated me because I had been using direct current therapeutically for many years. APS treatment produced rapid results on bruises, contusions, and wounds. It also affected inflammatory disease processes and improved general health and mental attitude. To my surprise, a single treatment often was sufficient to relieve a specific condition in a particular patient. In 1999, I wrote a book titled *Introducing Action Potential Currents* to assist patients and therapists using the APS device. I demonstrated APS therapy extensively in Israel, especially in pain clinics, and gave presentations with the late Professor Christiaan Barnard at an APS congress in Germany, where APS is used extensively. I also presented a seminar on APS (MDC) in Melbourne, Australia.

In addition, I have evaluated devices that use electric currents to treat sympathetically mediated pain, such as the U.S.-developed STS Dynatron, as well as electric-current treatments developed in Switzerland to strengthen weakened muscles. I have also worked extensively with magnetic and laser therapies. New treatments and devices involving electrical currents continue to be developed and researched, and I believe that many diseases and injuries will eventually be treated using these technologies.

There is another form of treatment that I wished I could offer all the patients who would benefit from it: warm water! I have often felt that if only a patient with a severely stiff and painful knee (or any other joint) could be placed in a warm pool, it would make all the difference in his or her treatment. Warm water relieves pain. My dream was realized in 2000 when I built an enclosed warm-water pool (93° F) and added a gym to my practice.

My current practice, The Pain Management Practice, is a noninterventional multidisciplinary pain-management practice specializing in physiotherapy, rehabilitation, psychotherapy, and dietary advice. For more information, see the Resources section at the back of the book. My professional journey leads me to continue focusing on pain management, as there is something new to learn in this fascinating field every day.

How This Book Can Help

Here are a few observations gleaned from my many years of treating chronic-pain patients: All patients who complain of pain actually have pain, although it may occasionally seem bizarre in its manifestation. Patients commonly name stress as the main factor that precipitated their crisis. I have found that a simple regimen of electrotherapy, acupuncture, relaxation, stress release, and exercise can bring great relief to patients. In some cases, patients have gained complete relief from their pain. In others, the pain changed and became more bearable, or the patient's coping strategies and quality of life improved. My conclusion is, therefore, that blocking pain, relieving anxiety, releasing emotions, and improving pain-free movements will help many patients on the road to pain relief. Treatments should, however, be tailored to the individual, and each person should be given the opportunity to try different treatments until one is found that helps his or her specific condition. Trial and error may seem haphazard, yet if it is applied systematically the right treatment will emerge and relief will be obtained. Some patients will respond to simple methods after many sophisticated, time-consuming, and expensive approaches have been tried, but others may require a "search party"!

This book aims to be a useful tool that can take the reader on a journey to pain relief by providing information and knowledge, suggesting better coping strategies, and teaching methods that empower patients to take control of their own pain. It may, hopefully, also obviate unnecessary tests and procedures.

The early part of the book discusses acute and chronic pain, with emphasis on factors that may increase pain and those that may improve the condition. Many of these factors depend on the patient. Therefore, it is essential for the patient to understand his or her own role in managing pain. Pain management is a team effort between patient and therapist, who work together to arrive at a satisfactory and, ideally, successful solution.

The later chapters provide information on acupuncture, electric currents, and exercise. Instruction is provided on managing pain using electric currents and other modalities, and advice is given on coping strategies and exercise techniques for specific situations.

I hope that through knowledge about their condition and about the range of therapeutic options available, patients will be transformed from passive recipients of treatment to empowered participants. Such a conversion can only help patients in their efforts to achieve the best possible result for their particular condition.

ACKNOWLEDGMENTS

I have many people to thank for helping me through my difficult but rewarding life journey. I would like to mention two very special individuals. The first is Professor and Master Leo Sebregts, who has been my mentor, teacher, and guide, and who has given me encouragement at every difficult turn and unfailing support with every achievement. The other special person is Professor Jesmond Birkhahn, who has extended my education in medicine and has given me faith and assurance that caring for and teaching patients, in fact, results in healing!

I would also like to take this opportunity to thank my best "teachers": my patients, who have taught me so much about the experience of pain.

CHAPTER 1

PAIN: THE NEVER-ENDING STORY

Pain is an unpleasant but often unavoidable part of the human experience. Sometimes people even experience pain from birth. Although never welcome, pain serves an essential function as a natural warning system that is critical for diagnosis and healing. We typically learn to accept pain due to its mostly transient nature.

Pain is a mystery. Although a minor injury, such as a simple bruise, contusion, or whiplash, may appear to heal, intense pain may be experienced months later for no apparent reason. On the other hand, some people who suffer traumatic injuries feel no pain at the time of the incident.

As we mature, we take various types of injury in stride, without fear or stress, because we understand their causes. Most injuries or cases of inflammation are uncomplicated and produce no need for concern because the healing process is apparent.

Acute Versus Chronic Pain

Acute pain is necessary. It serves as a warning that an injury has taken place. Acute pain produces the desire to be still and rest, especially during the initial period of discomfort. This limitation of activity may continue, to a certain degree, throughout the healing process. The immediate, general restraint of movement caused by a fracture, for example, preserves the bone ends until healing or medical intervention has taken place.

Pain that disappears after a short time is easily accepted. The problem is not acute pain, but rather chronic pain—pain that just never seems to go away. It has now been discovered that severe, acute pain that is experienced for even less than twenty-four hours can develop into a chronic-pain syndrome. It may seem terrifying that a patient could be predisposed to chronic pain within so short a period, yet it is also accepted that the key to preventing chronic pain is to *treat acute pain immediately.*

A chronic-pain condition is one in which pain usually persists longer than six weeks (or three months, according to some researchers). The normal period of healing in soft-tissue injuries is six weeks. By contrast, chronic pain may last for years, and in some patients it never truly disappears. We need to understand that the damage that occurs to the nervous system from severe pain often outlasts the actual injury; it is as if a telephone keeps ringing even though the call has long since been disconnected.

The most disturbing aspect of chronic pain is that it causes suffering. Pain may manifest as sharp, shooting, deeply aching, burning, spontaneous, and it is often unrelenting. It may present as a painful sensation at a mere touch (hyperesthesia, allodynia), which is an abnormal reaction.

When a patient has pain, it is important to eliminate serious health conditions such as cancers, tumors, and specific diseases requiring medical treatment as possible causes. To this end, all diseases and symptoms must *first* be evaluated in consultation with a doctor. This book provides specific information on obtaining rapid pain relief in the early stages of most conditions of chronic musculoskeletal or inflammatory joint pain *after* it has been shown that there is no cause for concern that further damage to the body may take place.

Chronic pain often has serious consequences for both body and mind and in some cases may never disappear completely. Because of this, many organizations, especially in Europe, have lobbied to have pain officially recognized as a syndrome. On the

Global Day Against Pain, held in October 2004, the International Association for the Study of Pain (IASP), an organization dedicated to improving knowledge in the field of pain management, stated that *chronic pain is now recognized as a disease.*

Our genetic history can predispose us to certain types of responses to injury or inflammation. Members of the same family may experience a similar type of pain upon being injured. Gender also plays a role.[1] Women tend to experience more chronic and recurrent pain conditions than men. Hormones, emotions, and social and cultural beliefs influence men and women differently with regard to pain. Most women tend to contain their emotions or life stresses within their bodies, which may then emanate as physical symptoms, and thus they tend to label stimuli as painful or to complain of spasms at different thresholds than do men. Women tend to report pain in the back, head, chest, abdomen, and face more often than do men. Men, on the other hand, learn to control or minimize their emotions when suffering from less obvious physical ailments, which may predispose some of them to conditions such as high blood pressure ("the silent killer") and its consequences, which may or may not be life threatening. It has also been noted that when treated with various pain-modulating drugs, men and women demonstrate differences in opioid function and in the molecular ability to bind to neuronal receptors.

Professor P. Prithvi Raj, a distinguished pain researcher and past president of the World Institute of Pain (a body of experts in pain management), once said, "You may never be able to take the pain out of the chronic-pain patient."[2] This is a moving reflection of the plight of many individuals suffering from chronic pain. It is also a comment on their treatment.

The Brain's Response to Pain

In a dangerous and traumatic situation, such as a shark bite, the brain produces a complex mixture of adrenaline and natural pain relievers (opioids) to enable us to escape and to protect us from the severe pain of the ordeal. This condition, commonly known as shock, may later cause severe physical and mental consequences. Some people feel no pain when they sustain serious injury during a sudden trauma; they experience complete temporary analgesia (relief of pain without loss of consciousness) during the event. And, as is well known, some people experience phantom pain and unpleasant sensations long after a limb (or even a tooth, breast, or other part of the body) has been amputated.

The first pain that we are aware of in a painful situation is usually an intense, sharp, fast pain, which may be followed by a slow, dull, aching, or even burning sensation. These different types of pain are due to different kinds of nerve fibers that convey information from the area of injury, called the periphery, to the spinal cord and then to the brain.

Simultaneous with the pain is the healing that takes place at this stage. The body is naturally armed with an immune system that moderates inflammation and fights infection. The body's endogenous (built-in) opioid mechanism produces various substances that not only relieve painful sensations but also facilitate the healing process. The immune system is complex and has an intimate relationship with the body's opioid pain-relief system. When the cells of the immune system are activated, the opioid receptors on all cells also become active. Opioid peptides appear to be dynamic signaling molecules that are produced within the immune system and are active regulators of an immune response. Recent studies of the interaction of opioids have indicated that opioid peptides are intimately involved with the immune system.[3] Thus, a strong immune system will have improved autogenic (self-producing) analgesic properties and abilities.

The brain (see Figure 1.1 on the next page) plays a role in the healing process. The injury or disease that created the damage in the individual is analyzed, in both the central scrutinizing center (cortex and limbic system) and the response-coordination center (thalamus, hypothalamus, pituitary) of the brain. This involves the thought processes as well as the emotions evoked by the situation, with a reaction taking place between the emotional and physiological responses to maintain homeostasis (the body's metabolic equilibrium).

Thought processes are affected by circumstances. If, for example, a person falls while rushing to an important meeting and injures the ankle ligaments, the stress of missing or being late to the meeting will affect the healing process. Or if a person is involved in a car accident, he or she may experience tremendous fear that the car will explode. Stress can cause some injuries, such as whiplash, to heal more slowly, or it can produce a prolonged period of pain and immobility before healing takes place. Pain stimulates healing, but stress slows healing.

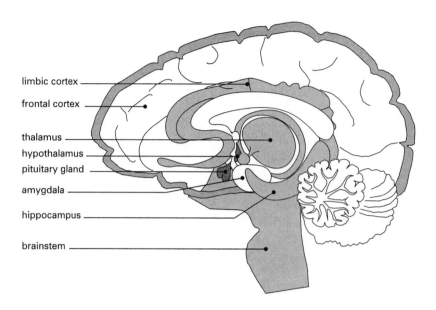

limbic cortex

frontal cortex

thalamus

hypothalamus

pituitary gland

amygdala

hippocampus

brainstem

FIGURE 1.1. The brain

See Figure 1.2. As explained by B.S. McEwen, "Perception of stress is influenced by experiences, genetics, and behavior. When the brain perceives an experience as stressful, physiologic and behavioral responses are initiated, leading to allostasis and adaptation. ['Allostasis' means stability or homeostasis through adaptation within the body.] Over time, allostatic load can accumulate, and the resulting overexposure to neural, endocrine, and immune stress mediators can have adverse effects on various organ systems, leading to disease."[4]

Past experiences also have an impact on our thoughts, which can promote or impede healing. For example, a person may fall on his or her knee and subsequently recall a friend sustaining a knee injury as a result of a similar type of fall. If the friend underwent a surgical procedure that failed, thinking about that may create increased and unnecessary anxiety and possibly delay healing.

People learn certain responses through their life experiences and sometimes react to a situation of pain with a reflex response rather than by means of a logical thought process. Pavlov famously conducted experiments in which he found that dogs who had come to associate the sound of a bell with food would salivate merely at the sound of a bell. Similarly, some people respond to pain with a reflex reaction, for example, holding their arm in a stiff position with the upper arm close to the torso, the elbow bent at ninety degrees, and the fingers in a clamped, flexed (bent) position. People also learn to associate chronic pain with certain forms of behavior or certain responses, such as lying down, grimacing, wincing, and groaning. This behavior will persist if positively rein-

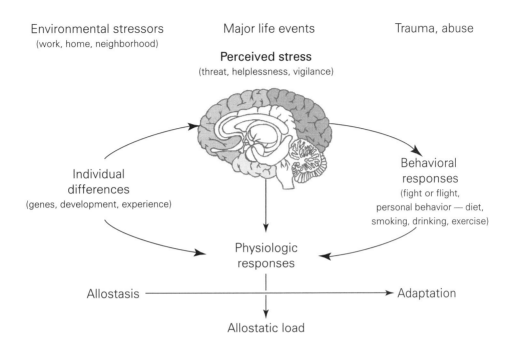

Environmental stressors
(work, home, neighborhood)

Major life events

Trauma, abuse

Perceived stress
(threat, helplessness, vigilance)

Individual
differences
(genes, development, experience)

Behavioral
responses
(fight or flight,
personal behavior — diet,
smoking, drinking, exercise)

Physiologic
responses

Allostasis ————————————————→ Adaptation

Allostatic load

FIGURE 1.2. The stress response and development of allostatic load.
Reprinted by permission from the *New England Journal of Medicine*. McEwen, B.S., "Protective and Damaging Effects of Stress Mediators," *New England Journal of Medicine* 338 (1998): 171–179. Copyright © 1998 Massachusetts Medical Society. All rights reserved.

forced, for example, by increased attention from others.

The Effects of Emotions and Thoughts on Pain

In 1994, the IASP defined pain as "an unpleasant sensory and emotional response associated with actual or *potential* tissue damage" (italics added).[5] This definition of pain, which has become accepted worldwide, indicates that even the thought of pain may have severe physiological and emotional consequences for the pain sufferer.

How we feel about our pain predictably produces one of two responses:

1. We may limit our movements in the specific area of the physical problem but still continue with our daily lives and heal quickly.

2. We may become disturbed by the injury, thereby forcing ourselves into a rigid posture, undertaking unaccustomed activity or movements, or adopting thought processes that may increase stress on the whole organism and delay healing.

The first group of people, those who tend not to be disturbed by their injury, can be called "responders." They are active, cope with pain well, and rarely use drugs or seek medical attention. The second group of people, those who become disturbed by their condition, are "nonresponders." They may become consumed by their pain, often resting all day, taking different medications, experiencing mood changes, and paying continuous visits to various doctors ("doctor shopping"). They often become anxious, depressed, and angry.

Emotions and memories have a powerful effect on pain. Significant emotive events are often unconsciously pushed into the background. Acknowledging and recognizing this connection may help release emotions and facilitate the healing process. The ability to bring these emotions and memories to the surface and then release them will, over time, reduce pain. In his books on back pain, John Sarno emphasizes that identifying the stress and other psychological factors in our lives and recognizing that the "tension-muscle" connection influences disease will help heal back pain and other conditions.[6]

Fear plays an enormous role in our response to pain. In fact, many people are more afraid of the consequences of pain than of the pain itself. People are afraid that more pain means more damage. In some instances, this actually is the case, such as when a fractured limb is moved before it is stabilized. In most painful conditions, however, this assumption is erroneous, yet such fear inhibits people from moving normally, causing stiffness and deconditioning, and affecting circulation in the local area and ultimately in the whole body. In this way, fear has a negative effect on the overall healing process. Inactivity often also increases muscle spasm, which increases pain and impedes healing. Movement is necessary for the body and mind to function normally. If movement is limited, bodily function and mental activity are reduced. (More about the relationship between pain and fear can be found in Chapter 2.) An interesting similarity to the fear of pain is the fear of falling, especially in the elderly. Once an older person falls, he or she can become nervous and afraid to move. This lack of mobility leads to decreased coordination and balance. Any experience that disturbs the psyche, such as pain, falling, or injury, will influence future thoughts and physical activities. After a fall, elderly people should continue with exercise and other suitable activities to strengthen the body, which is a more effective and better strategy for preventing future falls than avoidance of activity.

Emotions and the Body's Biochemistry

As a result of thoughts, emotions, previous experiences of self and others, and memories evoked by the effect of the injury or inflammation on the central processing center, reactions take place in the motor, autonomic, neuroendocrine, immune, and sensory systems. These reactions precipitate physiological responses that facilitate electrical activity within the cells and tissues and produce chemicals that either promote or prolong the healing process.

Emotional pain is similar to physical pain and creates depression, anxiety, and suffering. New studies have revealed that the same chemicals are released in our body with pain as with depression. Negative feelings about one's condition and one's pain produce a biochemical response. For example, negative thoughts may result in higher levels of cortisol and noradrenaline (which reduce the effect of endorphins), substance P (which increases pain), and catecholamines such as adrenaline and noradrenaline (which produce widespread effects including vasoconstriction, accelerated heart rate, and "enhancement of fear-related memory formation").[7] If a situation disturbs us, fear and distress may cause the constriction of nerves and the contraction of muscles, which can contribute to pain or disease.

The body's internal environment, therefore, affects the healing process. Negative influences that hinder healing include poor health, a sedentary lifestyle, an unhappy disposition, a weakened immune system, poor diet, and a previous injury to the same or another region of the body that may have required a long time to heal. Positive influences that promote healing include the maintenance of good health, exercise, a good diet, and psychological well-being.

The Effects of Pain on the Psyche

Just as our psychological state affects our experience of pain, the converse is also true. Chronic pain often produces unhelpful beliefs and thoughts. For example:

- ◆ "Getting older means more pain."
- ◆ "To complain of pain demonstrates a weak character."
- ◆ "My illness is getting worse."
- ◆ "I deserve to have pain."
- ◆ "I am being punished for past actions."

Chronic pain that continues after repeated unsuccessful treatment and long-term use of analgesics and other drugs can cause reduced activity, loss of employment, family stress, loss of control over circumstances, physical deterioration, and worst of all, feelings of helplessness, irritability, depression, anger, and fear. Most people with chronic pain do not consciously realize that pain can depress their spirits; they may only recognize a feeling of despair and helplessness without understanding that it results from their pain. Medication used for pain also often has side effects, such as constipation and lethargy. And sleeplessness, which is a prominent symptom in the chronic-pain patient, often leads to exhaustion.

Antidepressants, anticonvulsants, and other medicines are now being prescribed in addition to analgesics to influence and reduce chronic pain. These drugs alleviate pain when administered in dosages that are smaller than those normally used for treating depression and epilepsy.

Pain and Anger

Health-care professionals have historically observed that anger is a common emotion found in chronic-pain patients.[8] These patients may experience frustration, hostility, and aggression. In particular, feelings of frustration and hostility toward the medical profession may arise when relief is not obtained. New theories that have been put forth by leading pain scholars and scientists suggest that anger and its expression, or inhibition, play an important role in the development of chronic pain. Anger may influence the adaptation to the pain, the healing process, and the overall well-being of the individual. The cause-and-effect relationship between pain and anger is complex. According to Ephrem Fernandez, anger may precipitate pain, predispose an individual to pain, exacerbate pain, become a consequence of pain, or even perpetuate pain.[9]

Anger can manifest both internally and externally. J. W. Burns says that the internal expression of anger increases paraspinal (i.e., surrounding the spine) muscle activity and releases adrenaline, causing increased muscle spasm and sensitization of nerve endings.[10] Externally, anger may be directed at medical personnel, family members, and friends. Activities and interventions intended to reduce anger toward a person's circumstances will affect and improve chronic-pain conditions.

Another aspect of pain, ill health, misery, and even the process of dying is that we become angry with, and unloving of, *ourselves.* Many patients become untreatable or unreachable. The best treatment in the world cannot help patients who do not want to help themselves. When we are in severe pain, we tend to reject treatment and the love of all those providing us with care and support. We become arrogant, distant, and angry with those who appear "healthy" and who love us.

The Physiology of Pain

Chronic pain is not biologically useful because it is usually unrelated to ongoing tissue damage and may even be the result of an imperfectly healed injury. It may be poorly localized; that is, instead of being experienced in a small area of the body or a particular joint, it may cover a whole region or limb and may even spread to the opposite side of the body (mirror pain). A painful stimulus can actually do damage to the body.

Chronic pain usually relates to changes in pain receptors called nociceptors, which are unattached nerve endings of afferent (incoming to the central nervous system) sensory fibers. The afferent nerves from the painful region relay the intensity and type of noxious stimulus to the next level of fibers, which are situated behind the spinal cord in a collection of neural tissue called the dorsal root ganglion (see Figure 1.3). The painful nerve transmission enters the spinal cord and is subsequently relayed to other areas of the spinal cord, to the sympathetic nervous system, back to the original region of injury, and/or to the brain.

Figure 1.3 represents the pathway of the sensory nerves bringing information from the periphery inward to the spinal cord, passing through the dorsal root ganglion, and entering the spinal cord at the dorsal horn. It connects with neurons to form a loop that exits the spinal cord through the motor nerve root. A connection is also made to the sympathetic ganglia of the sympathetic nervous system along this pathway. Synapses occur in the spinal cord that connect with pathways (dorsal and spinothalamic tracts) from the dorsal horn to the upper levels of the central nervous system and brain.

The probable regions involved in chronic pain relate to the area of the earlier injury,

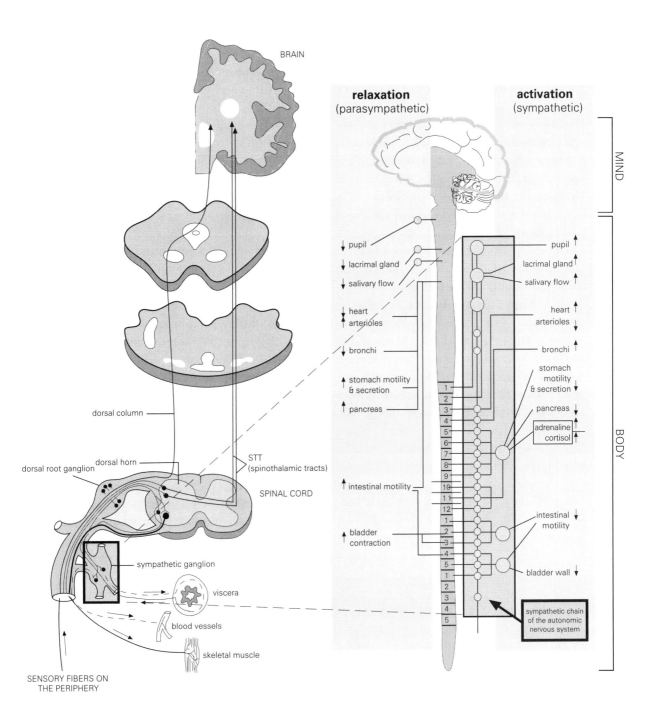

FIGURE 1.3. The periphery, spinal cord, and autonomic nervous system (ANS)

the dorsal root ganglion, the sympathetic chain of neurons (situated in front of the thoracic spinal column), the dorsal horn of the spinal cord, and several areas in the brain. The physical causes of pain are changes in the structure and function of this system, with electrical and biochemical changes taking place after the injury and sensitization of these areas. The body and brain function via electrical circuits and chemical substances. If there is a blockage in electrical transmission across the cell membranes or along a nerve fiber, or if chemicals are produced that increase inflammation and pain, the system (body and brain) will malfunction.

Although they are difficult to measure using standard medical technology such as X rays and blood tests, these chemical and electrical changes prevent the body from responding normally, including preventing the production or release of anti-inflammatory substances or pain-relieving opioids in adequate quantities. In some conditions, persistent changes in neurons produce muscle wasting and weakness, as well as changes in skin thickness, color, temperature, and circulation. These changes in the activity of sensory neurons are manifested as alterations of normal sensations.

"Rewiring" may also take place; painful stimulus can cause the normal electrical pathway from nerve endings to adapt, potentially repatterning the nervous system's connections in the dorsal horn of the spinal column, and producing electrical circuits that are overactive and spontaneously discharge, often causing sharp, paroxysmal, shooting, electric-shock pains. This may take place when growth buds called neuromas form on the damaged peripheral nerves. These tumors are benign (noncancerous) and usually self-limiting in size.

Unfortunately, pain begets pain. The more pain a patient experiences, the greater the likelihood of a general increase in muscle spasm, reduced breathing capacity and oxygen intake, increased activity from the sympathetic nervous system, and reduced circulation in the whole region, as well as reduced microcirculation in the local area. This increases the changes in the chemicals being released in the tissues, with more algogenic (pain-producing) substances being circulated.

An experiment on rats was mentioned at the World Institute of Pain Congress in 2000 in which each animal was restricted in a specially designed container so that only the head, tail, and feet were free during the experimental period. When these animals were killed, an increase of substance P was found in the spinal cord. Substance P, or neurokinin 1 receptor, is a peptide that increases circulation and swelling and boosts the release of histamine and serotonin, thus sensitizing nerve endings. It is found in areas of increased pain. The rats were not physically injured, yet the increased stress caused them to produce substance P. People with chronic pain are stressed due to their pain, and they produce substance P, which compounds the painful condition. Substance P has been implicated in many human diseases ranging from asthma to chronic bronchitis to inflammatory bowel disease to migraines.[11]

One study found that substance P introduced into brainstem nuclei increased breathing rates, whereas enkephalin (a naturally occurring pain-relieving neurotransmitter) decreased breathing rates.[12] Therefore, controlled breathing exercises may help patients who are in pain to reduce their levels of substance P, thus improving pain relief (see Chapter 3).

Chronic pain has serious consequences for the nervous system and can affect the whole body. Pain injures the local and central nerve supply by the constant barrage of impulses passing through the region. The autonomic nervous system responds to the stress of the pain by increasing blood pressure, heart and breathing rate, and cortisol levels. The response in these regions of the body stems from information relayed from three areas of the brain: the cortical area (thinking region), the thalamus (relay station for incoming/outgoing signals), and the hypothalamus and pituitary gland (hormonal and metabolic regulators). The latter two areas regulate hormones, metabolism, the autonomic nervous system, neurochemicals for pain control, and many other functions.

The autonomic nervous system (ANS) is important because it controls many organs and systems, including respiration, circulation, temperature regulation, metabolism, digestion, sweating, and endocrine secretion. The ANS is divided into two parts, the sympathetic nervous system (SNS) and the parasympathetic nervous system (PNS).

The SNS activates organs to prepare the body for fight or flight. It produces adrenaline and secretes norepinephrine directly into the bloodstream to help the body escape from difficult and frightening situations. Norepinephrine is a vasoconstrictor that also stimulates the adrenal gland to produce cortisol, the primary stress hormone. SNS activation results in temperature changes and the constriction of blood vessels. The skin may become flushed or sweaty and may develop goose pimples. The PNS, by contrast, stores and conserves energy by slowing the heart rate, enhancing digestion and food absorption, and emptying the bladder and bowels. It is responsible for the "relaxation response," which is the opposite of the fight-or-flight response.

The SNS and PNS work together to help maintain a functional balance in the nervous system, as both supply nerves to almost all the internal organs and other parts of the body. The SNS may become overactive when a patient is suffering from a pain condition or disease. The PNS helps to balance the SNS and may be activated for the control and reduction of pain, especially when the SNS becomes dysfunctional. The PNS may be enhanced or facilitated by closing the eyes, relaxation, visualization, and breathing exercises. (See Chapter 2 for more about the physiology of stress and the fight-or-flight response, and Chapter 3 for more about how to activate the PNS.)

Conditions That May Produce or Promote Chronic Pain

Chronic pain can result from a variety of conditions, some of which are listed below. Not every patient will necessarily produce any or all of these symptoms.

◆ Back pain in any area and from any nonmalignant cause

◆ Pain in any region that relates to malignancy (i.e., pain from cancer, which is usually a direct consequence of a tumor compressing tissue such as bone, blood vessels, and nerves)

◆ Pain from fractures due to injury, osteoporosis, or cancer

◆ Pain in the back after spinal surgery (known as "failed back syndrome")

◆ Inflammation related to arthritic damage to skin, soft tissues, joints, or bone

◆ Myofascial pain, in which tender and active regions (trigger points) in muscles become exquisitely sensitive, produce stiffness in joints, and stimulate sympathetic responses such as nausea and sweating; may be aggravated by stress

◆ Fibromyalgia, a complex condition of pain in designated, palpable fibrous tissues (particularly muscle fiber sheaths) that is associated with generalized muscular aching, stiffness, fatigue, and nonrestorative sleep; areas of pain that include the joints and muscles of the back, neck, ribs, chest, hips, knees, ankles, feet, shoulders, elbows, wrists, and hands; swelling; the feeling of "pins and needles"; and anxiety and depression may also be present

◆ Complex regional pain syndrome (CRPS; previously known as reflex sympathetic dystrophy), a condition that creates a dysfunction of the peripheral and central nervous system, in which pain, circulatory changes, and decreased mobility occur; usually affects the upper and lower limbs, but many patients with knee problems develop the condition, especially after surgery; if involvement of the central nervous system persists, CRPS may spread to the other side of the body or even envelop the whole body (see Chapter 10

for an in-depth discussion of treatment options for the pain of CRPS)

◆ Postherpetic neuropathy (a.k.a. shingles), a condition in which the herpes zoster virus attacks nerve endings, typically along a single dermatome (the body area served by a single spinal nerve) and only on one side of the body (unilateral). The trunk is most frequently affected, and shows a rectangular belt of rash from the spine around one side of the chest to the breastbone (sternum). The condition produces vesicles (small blisters) on the skin that become painful but eventually disappear, and the skin over the affected area continues to experience severe burning and tingling sensations

◆ Diabetic neuropathy, which can produce weakness, swelling, burning, and tingling sensations in the lower legs; other nerve endings may also be affected, for example, in the lumbosacral plexus and carpal tunnel; inflamed joints and poor circulation in the area of the damaged nerves may also occur

◆ Trigeminal neuralgia, in which the trigeminal nerve (a cranial nerve emanating from the brain that has three branches supplying the face) becomes diseased through local demyelination (loss of fatty tissue in the nerve sheath) of the trigeminal root; it may occur spontaneously and produce pain in the face, jaw, teeth, or head, as well as hypersensitivity to washing, chewing, teeth-brushing, or speaking; often accompanied by headaches and a stiff and painful cervical spine

◆ Headaches, including migraine, tension, or cluster headaches, or any persistent nonmalignant head pain

◆ Chronic venous insufficiency, which usually occurs in the legs and produces severe pain from blood vessels that are blocked or damaged by disease, injury, or postsurgical procedures; may cause swelling, discoloration, lack of blood supply, and an oxygen deficit in the surrounding tissues

◆ Phantom pain syndromes, which occur in a limb that has been removed, a tooth after dental procedures, a breast postmastectomy, or any amputated region of the body; may produce burning, sharp, or twinging electrical-shock pains, often with unusual and unpleasant sensations that can spread to other body areas

◆ Surgical incisions, which become very sensitive to the touch, producing spontaneous twinges, shocks of pain, and tingling sensations, due to damage to the skin nerves during the surgery

◆ Age-related degeneration of joints that is often of a musculoskeletal origin, producing stiffness and even headaches

◆ In the elderly, falls causing fractures and injured joints (falls are the leading cause of death in people older than sixty-five, according to the U.S. National Safety Council)

◆ Injury to the spinal cord, which often causes severe pain, usually at or above the level of injury; pain may take the form of spasm, burning, twinging, or shooting pain, which may spread into the paralyzed limbs

◆ Multiple sclerosis and other diseases that affect the central or peripheral nervous system; may cause spasm, burning, or shooting pain, and sensations in the head, spine, or limbs

◆ Stroke or head injury, which can cause severe, unrelenting pain in a paralyzed limb or in the affected side of the body ("central pain") as a result of thrombosis in the blood vessels of the brain; pain in the shoulder and arm, or the hip and leg, may occur due to severe contractures (abnormal and permanent muscle contractions) that develop as a result of constant reflex spasm; if the affected limbs are flaccid (hang limply) and are paralyzed, pain may occur from damaged or dislocated joints, lack of muscle support, and reduced circulation

◆ Iatrogenic injury (injury that occurs from medical procedures), such as venipuncture (for an IV drip), an overly tight immobilizing structure such as tourniquet or plaster of Paris, injections, spinal blocks, surgery, or any other medical intervention

◆ A viral attack on nerve roots or branches, which can produce a brachial neuralgia (acute spasmodic nerve pain)

◆ Mild sprain of a joint (often the ankle), contusions, or bruises in any region of the body

◆ Anterior knee pain caused by, for example, inflammation resulting from the lower surface of the patella rubbing on the femur (chondromalacia patella);

other areas in the knee joint may also become persistently painful, affecting the muscles surrounding the knee and manifesting in a rapid loss of strength, especially in the medial knee muscles (vastus medialis); this predisposes a patient to more pain because the muscular structures are providing inadequate support to the bone; the low back may also be compromised by poor walking patterns

◆ Damage from radiation to skin, muscle, and joints, mostly in the case of cancer patients undergoing radiotherapy

◆ Neurotoxicity (damage to the nervous system from a poison), which can produce severe burning pain in the limbs, spine, and head; neurotoxic poisons include lead, mercury, and even toxins in cigars (causing a condition known as Cuban neuropathy)

◆ Any pain, especially if neglected or prolonged

Treatment Options for Chronic Pain

Besides the administration of oral pain medications, many different procedures have been used to relieve discomfort:

◆ Local anaesthetic injection (lidocaine) into an area of pain

◆ Epidural and facet blocks (injection) into the spine

◆ Sympathetic blocks delivered by injection (usually phentolamine) into the sympathetic ganglia

◆ Sympathectomy: removal or destruction (via surgery, chemotherapy, or radio-

therapy) of the sympathetic ganglia involved in the pain

◆ Peripheral nerve blocks delivered by injection (usually lidocaine), or peripheral nerve stimulation (via an electrical stimulator implanted near the affected peripheral nerve)

◆ Implantation of a dorsal column (spinal cord) stimulator

◆ Regional blockade to the whole limb delivered by injection (via guanethedine or another substance)

◆ Burning or scarring nerves in the spine through the use of a radio frequency that produces a precisely controlled heat source

◆ Freezing nerves responsible for pain (cryoanalgesia)

◆ Neurolytic blockade with chemicals (e.g., glycerol) that are injected into specific regions of the brain or spine to destroy neurons responsible for pain

◆ In the past, deep brain stimulation via insertion of electrodes into regions such as the periaqueductal gray region, the thalamus, and the anterior cingulate gyrus; recently, greater success has been achieved through stimulation of the motor cortex on the surface of the brain

◆ Surgery, for example to remove a tumor or a damaged limb

Healing Requires a Change in Attitude

Pain does not have a fixed pathway that can be removed like a varicose vein, but is more like a transaction that takes place between the periphery and the central nervous system, involving different regions of the brain and producing an individualized response to pain.[13] One of the most important features of pain is that it is unique to and perceived differently by each individual.

A friend who has sustained an injury similar to yours may experience different pains and feel different emotions relating to the incident. The healing process and the time it takes may also be different. No other person can ever experience our pain! Pain can be likened to an individual's fingerprint; the source of the imprint for the whole body exists in the brain and is like a neurological signature.[14] This means that each person who experiences pain requires a specific analysis and understanding of the condition and situation.

Part of healing usually involves changing our *attitude* and our *perception* of the pain. Doing so is a progressive experience, and how we manage this process will facilitate the alleviation of pain or illness. It will also assist other natural processes, such as dying. When we're afflicted with pain, instead of turning on ourselves and on others, we need to accept the comfort, love, and healing provided to us. If we change our attitude, it opens the door to improved health, happiness, contentment, and acceptance. If we understand that our attitude and disposition and the emotions of stress and fear play an important role in our responses, we come to realize that we have more control over the situation and over our own healing than we previously thought possible.

CHAPTER 2

RESPONSES TO PAIN

A forty-four-year-old male fractured his left ankle in a motorcycle accident. The talus and lateral malleolus bones were screwed and plated, but the talus failed to heal properly (nonunion). Here is the patient's own description of his overall condition and state of mind after he had been on crutches and had worn a protective boot for a year:

> As the financial director of a medium-sized company, I felt the injury and walking on crutches had a major effect on my performance at work. I lost a lot of confidence in myself and felt very inferior. During presentations, I often stuttered and lost track of my thoughts. I now have felt a little of what people with permanent disabilities feel—tolerance is required, not sympathy. In my opinion, colleagues at work naturally adopted the law of the jungle: The weak must not survive; get better or get eaten.
>
> I was very disappointed in the doctors' perception and understanding of my pain. Many were very uncomfortable; they would look through my X rays but hardly interact with me about the reasons for and treatment of the pain. The prescription of over-the-counter painkillers is a good example. I felt the pain caused me to withdraw and lose interest in my family and other people. More importantly, it has left me with compassion for others whom I see and hear experiencing pain. With pain, it is difficult to be positive about one's chances of recovery. Remaining positive, to me, is a very important contributor to getting healed. I am surprised that many of the orthopedic surgeons I have seen did not recommend physiotherapy. I certainly would not like to contemplate what my ankle would have looked like without physio.

Despite enduring all the tests, medications, and interventions appropriate for their condition, many patients often continue to have pain symptoms for a long time.

It appears that "pain" poses a "question" that requires an "answer," but most of the time there are *no* answers or simple explanations because, in such conditions, pain can be invisible. It can exist when there is no tumor or blockage, when nothing can be found through an X ray or other scan, and when blood tests show no indication of where the pain is coming from.

The lack of a visible, palpable, physical source of pain is common in the chronic-pain patient. This is usually because the original problem has healed (even if imperfectly), leaving the patient with a derangement in the peripheral and central nervous system. An aberrant nervous system is not properly responsive to the normal treatments for pain.

As we saw in Chapter 1, pain affects the body at a physiological and psychological level and negatively influences the healing process. Constant pain has adverse consequences for both the endocrine and metabolic processes. It can affect sugar levels, the lungs (due to decreased oxygen), the kidneys (due to reduced elimination), and the heart (due to increased heartbeat and blood pressure). Neurologically, chronic pain may affect the reflex responses in the spine and brain—the nervous system's "memory" of pain—potentially creating hyperalgesia (increased responsiveness to pain) and central hyperexcitability (excess reactions in the spinal cord and brain). This type of situation is difficult to alleviate with standard medication and treatment.

Pain creates stress and tension throughout the body, including pressure on the nerves in the neck and back, with effects on the legs and arms.[1] The physical consequences are an increase in metabolites, local oxygen deficit, and widespread motor, sensory, and sympathetic activity (i.e., release of noradrenaline, which sensitizes nerve endings). Pain can cause increased respiration, which reduces chest expansion and decreases oxygen supply. Muscle spasm further increases stimulus at the site of the pain, by creating changes in microcirculation, local acidity (increasing pain), and pain substances.

The Pain Cycle

The pain cycle is a negative feedback loop that increases pain. Higher levels of pain lead to increased feelings of fear, helplessness, and anxiety, and to more sleep deprivation—which all increase the pain. The patient becomes more despondent and depressed as the pain continues, seemingly without abatement.

The aim of all treatment is to break this vicious cycle, especially by relieving the pain. Addressing the other aspects in this loop, such as fear, anxiety, and sleep deprivation, also contributes to breaking the cycle.

When pain becomes all-encompassing and relentless, it reduces the patient to a state of inertia, both mentally and physically. Relief from pain, even if only for a few hours, is as if a cloud has lifted, allowing the patient to see that there is hope that something may help. It is important to reassure the person that if the pain decreases, even if only for a short while, it is good news. The sufferer needs to know that as the treatment persists, this temporary abatement of pain can happen again, with increasing frequency, until the pain eventually subsides or leaves.

Therapy Can Be a Double-Edged Sword

During consultation and treatment, some patients may experience trauma at the hands of an unwitting doctor, physiotherapist, or other medical caregiver. Patients are often overtreated and overexamined. Many patients feel more pain after they have been "put through their paces" during the therapist's effort to determine the source or extent of the problem. Forcing movements through pain often increases pain; if pain is the syndrome, doing so may affect the disorder itself.

Often, a patient may experience more pain after a treatment, especially after physiotherapy. Such pain is referred to as "treatment soreness" and can actually decrease overall recovery time. When a treatment causes discomfort or pain that disappears shortly after the treatment, it is acceptable. There is nothing, however, to be gained from increased pain if it does not disappear shortly after treatment. Increased pain may lead to an overall upsurge in pain and could exacerbate the pain state itself.

Patients are not always given 1) the clear, understandable explanations about their problem and 2) the explanation about the procedure(s) required to assist the condition that would set their minds at ease. Communication between doctors and patients is often poor, with patients leaving the consultation with the impression that the doctor has failed to understand, believe, or listen to information about their problem.

Patients hang on *every word* spoken by their therapist and, more importantly, by their doctor. These words may either create

alarm or put patients' minds at rest. Creating stress or alarm fuels a fear of loss of control, of increased pain, and even of death. Proclamations by a medical professional that have a negative connotation can depress patients and cause their condition to deteriorate. Many patients often leave their therapist or doctor feeling more unsure, afraid, distressed, and worried about their condition than before the consultation or treatment. The words spoken to the patient should be reassuring, encouraging, kind, caring, helpful, and *positive.*

Doctor Shopping

The word "doctor" has its origins in the Latin word *docere,* which means "to teach." The main role of a doctor or medical professional is to explain the condition and the treatment to the patient, offer reassurance and relieve anxiety, and teach the patient how best to cope and help him- or herself heal. "Doctor shopping" is the term used to describe the activity of making constant visits to different doctors to try to find the answer to the pain.

Doctor shoppers believe that perhaps the next doctor will have the solution (medication and procedure) to "take the pain away." Some patients seem to be more relieved when a diagnosis (even if terminal) is made, because they feel that a diagnosis equals a solution. Patients believe that if they actually have a name for their condition, their doctor, family, or friends will not regard them as malingerers. Unfortunately, many doctors may feel obliged by a patient's desperation to investigate or operate when the best approach would have been to leave well enough alone and to analyze the situation from a multidisciplinary perspective. Many surgical operations performed "for pain" end up increasing pain and debilitation, and they may also weaken the bone and nerve structures, thus creating irreparable harm.

Medical Information on the Internet

Modern times have catapulted us into the era of the incredible World Wide Web, which provides information on every possible subject. While it is important and educational to have so much information at our fingertips, sometimes too much knowledge can be a dangerous thing! Often patients come to see me carrying screeds of information that they have accumulated about their condition from various websites. They may become deeply concerned about the possibilities that could occur or worried that the treatments that have "gone wrong" for others in their particular situation could happen to them.

My advice is to use the Internet to find out more about a particular condition, and then discuss the problem with a trusted clinician or therapist. Taking things into your own hands by relying completely upon what you find on the Internet can be deeply disturbing and can lead to the conclusion that nothing further can be done. The best approach is to select the advice and treatment that make you feel as if you are on the right track and that give you confidence, and then do as much as possible for yourself to improve your general health and state of mind. The most recent and scientific information on pain can be found on the website of the International Association for the Study of Pain, at www.iasp-pain.org.

Stress

Remember from Chapter 1 that pain can result in stress, and stress can increase pain. It is now acknowledged that to understand what stress does to the body we also need to understand its effects on the psyche. In the last fifty years much research has been done on the "stress response," and we are beginning to understand that the problems associated with stress result from a complicated interaction between the outside world and the body's capacity to manage potential threats. These complexities involve such seemingly disparate factors as heredity, childhood experience, diet, exercise, sleep patterns, the presence or absence of close relationships, income, social status, and the increase of normal stresses to the point that they psychologically overload the system.

The stress response is part of our survival mechanism—the "fight-or-flight" response. This mechanism facilitates escape from threatening or difficult situations as a result of automatically increased heart rate, blood pressure, and oxygen to the muscles to produce the energy required to take flight or stay and fight. The stress response also primes immune cells to rush to the site of a potential injury. Even a thought of danger or pain can initiate this reaction. After the danger, threat, or potential for pain is no longer imminent, the parasympathetic nervous system returns the physiology to a state of homeostasis/allostasis, or balance.

The autonomic nervous system is controlled by the hypothalamus, which is commonly known as the "master gland." The hypothalamus receives the message of danger from the brain and delivers a message through the nervous system to every other system of the body. The hypothalamus also signals the endocrine system to initiate the secretion of hormones, primarily adrenaline and cortisol, from the adrenal glands, which are positioned on top of the kidneys. These hormones flood the bloodstream and travel throughout the body to help create the ability to be more speedy and powerful.

Epinephrine (adrenaline) and norepinephrine (noradrenaline) are released into the bloodstream from the inner part of the adrenal gland, known as the adrenal medulla. Cortisol, a key stress hormone, is released from the outer part of the adrenal gland, known as the adrenal cortex. Together, these hormones flood every cell in the body with the specific message to prepare for fight or flight.

When stress persists for too long or becomes too severe, the normal protective mechanisms become overburdened, and the feedback process goes out of control, with resultant damage to the whole system. This overburdening has been shown to weaken the immune system, strain the heart, damage memory cells in the brain, and even deposit fat at the waist instead of the hips and buttocks (a risk factor for heart disease, cancer, diabetes, and many other diseases). At the first sign of danger, the hippocampus and the amygdala are alerted. High levels of cortisol can shrink nerve cells in the hippocampus and even curtail the production of new hippocampus neurons. These changes are also associated with aging, memory problems, posttraumatic stress disorder, and depression.[2,3]

In the United States, observations of people exposed to stressful events demonstrated that 90 percent of patients presenting with a life-threatening disease had experienced a disturbing and traumatic event eighteen months to two years prior to developing the condition. According to Steven Locke, of Harvard University, natural-killer-cell activity (an important component of the immune system) decreases during periods of heightened life changes that are accompanied by severe emotional distress. People going through life changes but who experience less emotional distress have normal natural-killer-cell activity.[4] Events including the loss of a relative, divorce, or other trauma can trigger illness. Many of my patients who suffer chronic low-back pain have mentioned similar events that occurred in their lives before their back problems developed.

Fear Avoidance

Fear avoidance implies avoidance of activities that may increase pain when there is actual pain but no active pathology. Unfortunately, lack of activity will worsen the condition, negatively affect the local circulation, and decondition the whole body. The patient learns to avoid the activity almost as a reflex response, instead of as the result of a logical plan of action. Once avoided, the activity will become very difficult to execute and ultimately will produce increased pain. For example, if a finger is held in one position for an hour, it will become very painful to move again, due to changes in the circulation and nerve endings. Avoiding a harmless activity becomes ingrained, and that avoidance will remain long after the healing process has actually taken place, thus producing stiffness, reduced fitness, and diminished ability to perform the task. This may eventually lead to disuse, pain, and hypersensitivity.

If an activity is very painful to execute, methods can be found in a nonpainful and supportive environment, such as in water, to reduce pain during the activity. This topic is discussed in "Coping Skills," Chapter 12.

Fear Affects Beliefs

In Chapter 1 we began to examine the connections between emotions, thoughts, and pain. Beliefs—about oneself, one's health, and one's life—are inescapably entwined in these interactions. When there is no light at the end of the tunnel, patients begin to believe the following:

◆ That they have no personal control over their pain or life

◆ That pain is going to disable them forever—"I am going to end up in a wheelchair"

◆ That pain means there is further damage

◆ That if they become distressed by emotional events, it may increase their pain—"Don't upset me or my pain will get worse"

◆ That they will require a large quantity of medication to relieve the pain, and that medication may be necessary for the rest of their lives

◆ That a medical cure exists to "take my pain away"

◆ That they will never get better, that there is no hope, and that there is no solution to their problem—and never will be!

All of these considerations[5] produce a person who has reasons to

◆ be helped by others (i.e., avoid taking responsibility)

◆ stay at home from work

◆ give up social responsibilities

◆ claim worker's compensation

◆ lose independence

◆ lose self-control

◆ have permission to have the pain

◆ take drugs/medication

◆ sleep all day, stay awake all night

◆ increase weight, drink alcohol

◆ become overactive when the pain eases, or do nothing when the pain returns/gets worse

Patients who avoid activities because of the fear of pain will become even more fearful of the pain, increasingly avoid *all* painful experiences, become physically unfit, become increasingly disabled, and, worst of all, be unable to be objective when measuring their own pain.

By constantly focusing on the pain and the damaged region of the body, the patient's memory of pain will become worse. He or she will become more fearful and anxious about the pain. Hypervigilance may set in, with the patient expecting the pain, watching for any increase or decrease in pain, and becoming overly concerned with the importance or value of any perceived increase or decrease in pain. Eventually, nothing else will be of any importance to the patient except *the pain!* This ingrains pain into the electrical and chemical memory and can be likened to travelling on a dirt road: If the road is well travelled it becomes a deep indentation, but if it is less travelled it could disappear.

Worry

Patients often feel that "if I just knew what was wrong," they could cope much better with their problem. They worry about worst-case scenarios and long for a diagnosis when they don't have one.

If pain itself is the actual syndrome or disease process, then it is safe to eliminate the pain because it does not exist to protect us from anything. Many seemingly unrelated conditions disappear once the pain has been relieved. This is often clearly demonstrated in patients with an acute, recent complex regional pain syndrome (CRPS) where, once the pain has been relieved, all the other symptoms of swelling, skin discoloration, temperature changes, and stiffness also vanish. It may be postulated that CRPS is a unique example, but, in my experience, many patients with back pain, or pain in other areas, have also achieved relief of symptoms after removal of pain. I believe that many more patients have conditions that can be relieved by elimination of the pain (after all other diagnoses are excluded).

It is often true that once we understand the problem (i.e., by receiving a diagnosis), a sigh of relief flows through us, we accept the situation, and we just get on with it. Chronic pain teaches us, however, that we have to learn to accept a "nondiagnosis" as a *positive* prognosis and a sign that the condition is, in essence, nonmalignant and nonthreatening.

Chronic pain also helps us begin to understand that, if there is no other explanation, the pain probably arises from a derangement in the nervous system and/or from stress and muscle spasm, which produce the "stress-tension effect." In such cases, new approaches in treatment must be taken to change the situation by blocking the pain, reducing pressure on the nerves, and relaxing and stretching the muscles, thereby achieving relief, control, and management of the pain.

Patients often become fearful that their condition is serious, especially when they have received a diagnosis that sounds alarming. However, being diagnosed with degenerative disc disease, crumbling discs, herniated discs, or pinched nerves does not necessarily mean a patient has the condition in its worst manifestation. The solution is to become less anxious and fearful about the condition, acknowledge life stresses, learn relaxation techniques, and increase exercises that stretch the tight muscles and strengthen and support the weak regions of the body as well as the specific sites of discomfort.

It is good news to know that our condition is not serious and can be treated! It means, at least, that we are not going to die from the pain. Now we have to find ways to *live* with it.

CHAPTER 3

PATIENT, HEAL THYSELF

No patient should suffer pain in silence. People are entitled to have their pain taken seriously. As mentioned, pain is now recognized as a syndrome and can become the disease itself. No patient should suffer because his or her pain has not been adequately relieved.

You—the patient—have the *right* to seek relief from pain. You may have to learn to adapt to some pain, but you have the right to request and find relief from bothersome, severe, or intolerable chronic pain. Every patient with complaints of pain is entitled to be *believed* and *respected,* and adequate medication or treatment should be offered or administered to relieve pain and suffering.

> You have the right *not* to remain silent.

Many patients have experienced unusual or bizarre pain and sensations that are now accepted as having been caused by an aberration in the nervous system. Many patients have been misunderstood by their medical professionals, both doctors and therapists, because their pain did not "fit" a standard diagnosis, outlasted the healing process, or produced "unnatural symptoms."

If pain is not relieved by simple analgesics (pain killers), or if it lasts longer than expected, consult your doctor, who may prescribe medication or treatment for pain relief. If relief is not forthcoming, you may be referred to a pain specialist or clinic, where you will meet with a group of health professionals who have an understanding of the problems encountered by people who experience unrelieved pain.

Most pain clinics offer a multidisciplinary approach because it is now being increasingly recognized that chronic pain has a serious effect on many different aspects of life. As you've seen, pain involves emotions as well as physical problems.

Your Rights as a Pain Patient

Every pain patient is entitled to be attended by *caring* and *listening* professionals. A study performed in England and published in the *British Medical Journal* compared two groups of physicians utilizing a similar therapy for a similar illness. Sympathetic, caring physicians carefully listened to patients and then treated the first group. "Detached" physicians, who merely administered the treatment, treated a control group. The result was not surprising: The first group responded substantially better than the control group, indicating that patients respond best when given the full attention and care of the medical attendant.[1]

There are a number of requisites in the interaction between patient and therapist that facilitate a positive treatment outcome. "Positive" here means that the effect readily demonstrates improved pain control and/or relief and a sense of achievement. These requisites include the following:

1. Patients are entitled to an *explanation* about their condition and treatment. This type of communication should continue throughout every interaction between patient and therapist or doctor.

2. The patient should frequently be reassured, because satisfaction and contentment with a therapy is the *key* factor in promoting a positive outcome.

3. Throughout treatment, therapists and doctors should constantly communicate and demonstrate the progress and improvement achieved by the patient, because "seeing is believing." When a patient has *proof* that something has happened (e.g., his or her movements are more flexible), realization dawns that there actually has been some improvement. Often, patients do not believe that any improvement has taken place until some aspect of progress is demonstrated to them. For instance, a knee that was stiff can now move into flexion, or a hand with previously inflexible fingers is now able to close and make a fist.

4. Every patient who succeeds should be *praised* for his or her achievement. Successfully getting better is the achievement of the patient, not of the therapist. The therapist can offer treatment, but the patient has to go through the motions, repeat the exercises, and make all the necessary effort for progress to be attained.

The More You Do, the More You Can Do

If a patient experiences severe pain and is therefore unable to function normally, he or she may be overcome with depression and inertia. However, this does not have to be so, as the following case study demonstrates:

MALE, AGE SIXTY-NINE

Diagnosis: painful lumbosacral diabetic neuropathy since 2001. Electrical-shock pain down the leg, severe back pain, painful knee and leg, pain spreading to the opposite side, unable to walk without crutches

This patient, a lawyer, had severe pain and hyperesthesia in his right leg, from the groin to the knee. The low back on his right side was constantly and extremely painful, his right leg was becoming weak, and he had to use a crutch to walk. The pain was intolerable and he became severely debilitated.

For many months, this patient was unable to work or socialize, due to pain. He felt that he was unable to perform normally in society and began to retreat, avoiding any activity that he believed was impossible due to the enormity of the pain. Physical movement was difficult, and his voice became tired and weak.

He commenced physiotherapeutic pain control in October 2002 and was encouraged to continue working. He experienced positive results. "I forced myself to make an effort to work and to interact normally within my family," he said. He found that the pain became less obtrusive, and he was eventually able to cope with a normal working day and lifestyle. Allowing himself to return to work and becoming involved in active therapy provided a "distraction" that enabled the patient to focus on other activities rather than pain, which, in turn, began to diminish in its importance and effect. He had greatly improved by December 2002, just two months later.

Knowledge Is Power

A patient will best be served by analyzing the situation and examining two factors:

1. How did this problem begin? What happened to create this pain?

2. How you feel now? What is the status of the painful part of the body?

Once this analysis has been performed and a logical explanation for the problem has been found, the patient can begin to accept the problem and its consequences. This facilitates healing and releases stressful emotions related to the pain.

If some degree of denial occurs, however, and the problem is ignored or becomes buried within the subconscious mind, the patient may forget the cause and its effect. If the problem persists, doubts about the true nature of the problem may arise. This can generate questions based on fear and anxiety:

◆ Why do I have this pain?

◆ Am I becoming really ill?

◆ Will I ever get better?

◆ What is happening to me?

By contrast, as long as a condition is not frightening and the patient understands and accepts it, the process of healing can occur unhampered by stress, anxiety, and fear. Even if a condition becomes persistent, if a patient accepts its existence, he or she can prepare to live amicably with the difficulties it presents.

An early diagnosis is, therefore, of utmost importance.

The earlier the diagnosis is made, the sooner the correct treatment can begin. If the patient receives reassurance from the doctor in the beginning that the condition is benign, or that the problem emanates from a local injury, from tension involving the muscles of the spine due to life's stresses, and/or from poor posture, and that only minimal physiotherapy and increased exercise will be required to alleviate the problem, the patient will be more at ease.

Narrative Medicine

In addition to the correct treatment for pain, a personal connection with the caregiver, therapist, or clinician is required for true healing. The patient has an emotional effect on the therapist, which in turn produces a healing connection or response for the patient. The intersubjective space between patient and therapist is the setting of care and attention, and this enables the patient to fully represent him- or herself.

Patients need to be able to tell their whole predicament (life story). This is true because the source of chronic pain can be complex past trauma that is knowable only through telling. Allowing patients to explore the larger context of their pain bears witness to their suffering. Narrative medicine helps the patient to draw the picture of his or her condition through words and emotions, including loss, trauma, the plot of the story, and many other aspects. It also helps to define the future and gives hope to the patient.[2] According to University of Calgary sociologist Arthur Frank, "Health-care workers who bring a sense of narrative to bear have transformative effects." Rita Charon, M.D., a physician and director of the narrative medicine program at Columbia University, advises the therapist to ask, "Tell me about your health, your body, and your life."

The following anecdotal story from Dr. Charon's book *Narrative Medicine: Honoring the Stories of Illness* tells of these profound effects on one of her patients, a thirty-six-year-old man with back pain who had come to see her for the first time.

As his new internist, I tell him, "I have to learn as much as I can about your health—tell me about your health, your body, and your life." I do not interrupt the man with pesky questions, I listen in an analytical way as if he were a charac-

ter giving a soliloquy. I listen not only for content of his narrative but for form, its temporal course, its images, its associated subplots, its silences, where he chooses to begin in telling of himself, how he sequences symptoms with other life events. After a few minutes he stops talking and starts weeping. I ask why he is crying.

He says, "No one has ever let me do this before."[3]

This "telling and listening" process improves the capacity of the clinician to recognize, absorb, interpret, and be moved by stories of illness. It also deepens the clinician's attention to the patient. It is another healing tool that can be used to help patients with pain or any other condition.

Research Findings on Pain and Exercise

To function optimally, the body needs to move and maintain its correct alignment. This is assisted by

◆ analyzing the best method to support the body for the particular occupation or sport

◆ doing exercises that stretch tight structures (usually the pectoralis and hamstring muscles)

◆ strengthening weak muscles (commonly the abdominals and back muscles)

The key factor in healing is to *keep moving!* The body is designed to move. If movement is restricted, reduced circulation occurs in the local region of damage and eventually leads to deconditioning in the whole body.

The following are some important research findings regarding the effects of exercise on pain:

- Pain relief may occur with high-intensity exercise.[4] Reaching 60 percent of maximum oxygen absorption is required to increase beta-endorphins in subjects without pain.[5] Many patients who are in pain cannot reach these vigorous exercise states to achieve beta-endorphin release, yet still experience pain relief from exercise, due to another type of nonopioid neurotransmitter release.[6] This may be due, in part, to the fact that *pain perception is altered after exercise*, probably via nonopioid mechanisms.[7,8]

- Both exercise and acupuncture produce rhythmic discharges in nerve fibers and cause the release of endogenous neurotransmitters.[9]

- Pain relief is dependent on exercise duration, regularity, and, in the case of water exercises, water temperature. Exercising in warm water relieves pain, but exercising in cold water does not.[10]

- Exercise has antidepressive effects.[11]

- Exercise may modify pain perceptions by enhancing psychological well-being.[12]

- Group exercise may affect pain perception via the added factor of socialization, including the aspect of distraction.[13]

In short, exercise relieves pain. However, most chronic-pain patients are afraid to exercise because they fear it will increase their pain. This fear is especially strong in cases when even a small movement may be painful.

This difficulty can be overcome in various ways:

- Exercise in *warm* water, either in the bath or in a heated pool.

- Start with *small* movements that do not increase pain, even without immersion in water.

- Remember that if pain increases during the exercise but disappears afterwards, that particular exercise will not harm you or exacerbate the painful condition.

- Exercise all the *nonpainful* areas of the body.

- Start with a *graded* exercise program, where minimal pain may occur. If this pain is easily managed, then the exercise is acceptable.

- *Expose* the body to some small discomfort in order to progress, but not so much that it increases the pain after the exercise.

- Increase general *fitness*.

- Walking and swimming are the easiest exercises to participate in, especially if you are extremely debilitated.

Tips for Overcoming Postural Problems That Could Be Created by Sitting at a Desk

The body has to be protected from poor posture and the injuries that can result from it. Activities that occupy our daily lives involve work, play, and relaxation. If these activities take place with a poor posture (one that fails to keep the body in correct alignment), injuries and strain of joints, muscles, and ligaments will persist, eventually creating pain, muscle spasm, and deformity.

Bad posture is typical of working at a desk, especially at a computer, for long periods of time while remaining physically inactive. Most people spend more time sitting when working and at leisure than in any other posture. Many back problems are compounded by long hours of sitting, especially in front of a computer. By concentrating on their work using only the eyes, head, and neck, people may be neglecting what is occurring in the rest of the spine.

Correct seating prevents muscle fatigue and wasted muscular effort. However, most people do not have the opportunity to select the correct chair for their height, weight, and posture, and for the specific tasks they perform. Thus, they have to adapt to many different seating positions.

There is no ideal chair for all people! Here are some suggestions to improve the ergonomics of sitting (see Figure 3.1):

- If the chair has arms, make sure they are correctly adjusted for height, so that the shoulders are relaxed and not hunched or raised when resting on the arms.

- Push your hips as far back as they can go in the seat of the chair.

- The chair height should allow your feet to be planted firmly on the ground or a footrest, with the seat pan set to ninety degrees or slightly more than that in relation to the seat back. If the angle

between the chair's seat and back is less than ninety degrees, the low back tends to slump or lose its normal arch (lordosis) or curve unless supported. If the seat angle is greater than ninety degrees, the back retains the lordosis, decreases stress on discs that are compressed when sitting for prolonged periods, and decreases the angle of hip flexion, which may be more comfortable for patients with osteoarthritis of the hip joint. However if the angle is too steep (i.e., much greater than ninety degrees), then an increased arch or curve could strain the back of a person who does not have a normal lumbar curve (due to genetics, injury, or disease), potentially stressing joints, discs, and nerves in the lumbar spine.

- The ideal chair has a lumbar support to fully support the lumbar arch. If the chair has no lumbar support, use a rolled up towel or cushion to improve back support. The suggested angle for the back rest of the chair is 100–110 degrees. This relaxes muscles, maintains the normal curvature in the back, and reduces disc pressure. The lumbar support should extend to maintain the support in the upper to mid-thoracic spine, allowing this area to rest in neutral or slight flexion (forward curve) depending on the posture of the individual. The support should change its shape from one supporting the arch in the low back to a forward curve for the upper back.

- The correct lumbar thoracic support will affect the head position and will help

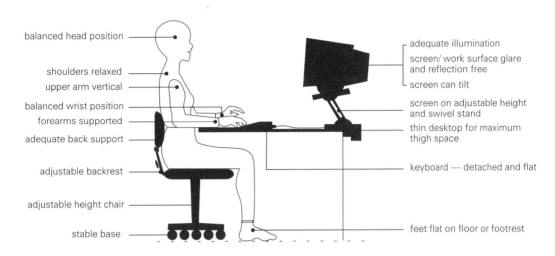

FIGURE 3.1. Correct sitting posture and correct chair positioning

the head to remain in an erect and neutral position, preventing compression on the posterior joints of the cervical and upper thoracic joints.

◆ The seat pan should not be too deep, as this encourages slumping of the lumbar spine and prevents the support from being maintained against the spine as the person has to move away from the backrest of the chair in order to reach the desk. It may also compress nerves or even the blood supply in the back of the legs and cause pain or discomfort.

◆ There should be no obstructions under the desk to prevent moving the chair close enough to be able to sit back in it and still reach the work tasks easily.

◆ When sitting at a computer, pull up close to the keyboard and position the keyboard in front of the computer screen, directly in front of you. The vision should be easily maintained without overextending the neck (moving the head upward and forward) to improve sight of the screen. The screen height and/or angle must also facilitate good vision. Ideally the eyes should be able to look straight ahead, maintaining an erect position of the neck (cervical spine), and then with a slight nodding movement of the head, the eyes should be able to move from the top of the screen downwards or around the screen. This will facilitate a slight arching (extension) and bending (flexion) of the neck.

Many chairs have an adjustable height and seat back. It is advisable to consider all of the above when adjusting the chair for your own comfort and efficiency at work. The seat pan should be fixed for stability and not move constantly as you work; although this does exercise the back muscles, over prolonged periods it may cause fatigue. If your job requires sitting at the desk or computer all day, you should make efforts to change your posture and do specific exercises. For example, take short one- to two-minute stretch breaks every twenty minutes; after an hour of work, take a break for at least five minutes to move around in order to prevent fatigue, muscle ache, and nerve compression. See Chapter 11 for descriptions of exercises to perform while sitting.

Oversensitivity to Pain with Exercise

This is a difficult subject to broach, because it applies to people who may perform the first movement of an exercise, feel pain, throw their hands up in fear and horror, and refuse to repeat the movement. You need to understand that there is "good" pain and "bad" pain.

A "good" momentary pain will be produced when stretching the ligament or muscle and will disappear after a short while. Persevering with this exercise and discomfort will actually improve the movement and decrease the pain—it is like nudging the pain then stepping back and nudging it again until more exercises can be performed without pain. Work around and with the pain!

A "bad" pain is one that does not go away after exercise, and if this is the case, the movement that causes the pain should be avoided. Yet, it is still important to push the body in the nonpainful areas, because a general improvement in circulation assists the injured region in becoming less sensitive.

Increase exercise step-by-step. Here is a suggested regimen for increasing your fitness if you are debilitated by pain:

- Walk from your front door outward bound for five minutes.

- Return the distance home within four minutes.

- Repeat daily for one week, until this exercise is performed easily.

- Increase the walking time to ten minutes outward bound and nine minutes to get home for the next week, until this exercise is performed with ease.

- Eventually increase the walking time to between twenty and thirty minutes outward bound and between nineteen and twenty-nine minutes to get home.

- Design your own challenges until fitness is achieved, strength is gained, and pain has decreased.

The primary aim is to reduce the fear of movement and exercise, build confidence in your ability to move, develop control of your body, obtain pain relief, and learn to *pace* yourself. Pacing is necessary because the most natural thing to do when pain feels better is to try and do everything that was impossible when you experienced severe pain. You may decide to clean the whole house, because you haven't cleaned for months, or do a month's grocery shopping in case the pain returns and you become housebound once again. That is a *big* mistake! The so-called overactivity/underactivity cycle can lead to a severe setback, and once again to the fear of trying to be "normal."

I suggest that smaller goals be attempted first, until you learn which activities may irritate your condition. Then, find ways to break these activities down into even smaller components, until the full activity is more easily achievable. It may be useful to associate the activity with a pleasant experience, such as meeting a friend for coffee once the shopping has been completed, which also provides an opportunity to rest and regain strength. It takes patience and perseverance, but success makes the achievement worthwhile. Gaining control and improving the quality of life are the rewards of learning to exercise with pain.

The Role of Laughter

Laughter is by definition healthy.

— Doris Lessing

Many patients with chronic pain demonstrate a sense of humor about their condition. Such patients inform me that it helps to have a sense of humor while coping with pain or other problems. Laughter can provide power over life's circumstances. It gives a different perspective on our problems, helping us to become detached from the problem, feel protected, and develop a feeling of control. Once we have control over our situation (pain), we have a greater sense of power and achievement. Many films and books have been written about humor and healing. The book *Humor Therapy* illustrates the use of humor in dealing with cancer, psychosomatic diseases, mental disorders, crime, and interpersonal and sexual relationships.[14] The movie *Patch Adams* told the true-life story of a doctor who believed in healing patients, even cancer patients, with laughter. Hospital researchers in the United States are now studying humor-intervention programs. Some hospitals now use a humor television channel to help improve patients' attitudes and healing.

Researchers at the State University of New York found that immune activity (salivary immunoglobulin, or IgA, levels) was lower on days of negative mood and higher on days of positive mood. A positive mood was measured by the amount of laughter. Studies at the Western New England College found that people showed an increased immune activity (e.g., interferon-expressing T cells and natural-killer cells were activated) after viewing a funny video.[15] Herbert Lefcourt, a psychologist at the University of Waterloo, in Canada, found that subjects who tested strongly for appreciation and utilization of humor had higher levels of immune substances after viewing a funny video than subjects who tested weakly.[16]

There is consensus among researchers that laughter

- lowers blood pressure
- reduces stress hormones (e.g., cortisol)
- strengthens the immune system
- triggers the release of endorphins

In her book *Laughing Matters,* Maria Funes states that the physiology of laughter affords many benefits:[17]

- Tears in the eyes contain more interferon, a molecule that is the first line of defense against certain viral and bacterial infections.
- Tears from laughter are a result of happiness, and tears from sadness are a release of the emotions, both of which are beneficial to the patient.
- Laughter produces higher levels of antibodies in the mouth, indicating enhanced immune function.

◆ Laughter helps the brain and body produce beta-endorphins, the internal opiates that help us relax and that reduce pain.

◆ Laughter reduces the production of stress hormones by the adrenal glands. For instance, cortisol levels increase in an unhealthy way during stress but decrease significantly with laughter.

◆ Blood pressure increases during laughter and drops below resting levels afterward.

◆ Laughter reduces muscle tension.

◆ Air is expelled rapidly from the lungs during a good chuckle, thus thoroughly oxygenating the body. This improves thought processes and aerobic fitness.

◆ Laughter's anti-inflammatory effect on the joints and bones can reduce inflammation and relieve pain in arthritic conditions (most arthritis begins with inflammation.) The immune stimulation from humor also makes connective tissues more resistant to inflammation in the first place.

The connection between natural pain relief from opiates (endogenous endorphins) and the immune system has now been solidified. Patients with strong immune systems have more effective pain-relieving mechanisms, and patients with strong pain-relieving mechanisms are healthier and better able to combat infection.

Patients with chronic pain should seek out situations and activities that bring joy, happiness and laughter into their lives in order to strengthen their system, uplift their spirits, and reduce the depression, anxiety, and fear associated with pain.

Breathing

A patient who has severe pain often develops distress when breathing. Breathing becomes shallow and light as the pain becomes stronger, causing less oxygen to reach all the cells of the body. This does not help pain—in fact, it may increase discomfort and add to suffering.

All living cells of the body require oxygen and produce carbon dioxide. The respiratory system allows oxygen from the air to enter the blood in the lungs and carbon dioxide to leave the blood and enter the air in the lungs. Shallow breathing does not allow sufficient oxygen to enter the lungs, nor does it eliminate sufficient carbon dioxide from the body.

An interesting study, mentioned in Chapter 1, demonstrated that when substance P (neurokinin 1 receptor antagonist) is injected into the brainstem it increases the frequency of respiration (breathing) by acting directly on certain neurons (pre-Bötzinger brainstem complex).[18] As we now know, substance P increases pain. An increase in pain will, therefore, increase the breathing rate and result in less oxygenation. In contrast, when enkephalin (a pain-relieving neurotransmitter) was injected into the same area of the brain, the breathing rate decreased and oxygenation increased. Researchers concluded that controlled, patterned breathing offers an effective nonpharmacological method for alleviating pain in both early and sustained pain.

It seems to be instinctive and part of our autonomic program that, a result of stress, fright, shock, and pain, we alter our respiration by breathing faster, which effectively reduces oxygen and increases carbon dioxide levels. However, we also have the natural ability to reduce our breathing rate, thus increasing oxygen intake and reducing carbon dioxide levels, which helps healing. Furthermore, breathing slower activates the parasympathetic nervous system. During parasympathetic activity (general relaxation) we are quiet and calm, and the body regenerates and restores for future activity. Some women may recall the breathing exercises taught in the 1970s (the Lamaze method) to alleviate pain in childbirth. We may have been admonished to "Breathe! Breathe!" during an uncomfortable procedure, because it is a known fact that breathing deeply relieves discomfort and that the distraction provided by the breathing exercise relieves pain.

The Role of the Parasympathetic Nervous System (PNS)

As mentioned, the physiological effect of deep, calm breathing is to stimulate the parasympathetic branch of the autonomic nervous system. This is the opposite of the action of the sympathetic nervous system, which produces the flight-or-fight response. The PNS is the "rest-repose" system and produces the "relaxation response" (see the next page); it is the great balancer of the body's automatic systems.

Activate the PNS by practicing some or all of the following techniques:

- Deep, slow, relaxed breathing
- Relaxation
- Closing the eyes
- Visualization

- Postural correction
- Midday rest
- Exercise

Therapists can stimulate the PNS by

- mobilizing the spine at the thoracic region, which includes all twelve thoracic vertebrae and their connection with the twelve ribs (the costovertebral joints)

- stretching neural tissue by moving the limbs, head, or both simultaneously, so that sensory and motor nerves are stretched as well as joints and muscles. All nerves are attached to the spinal cord (an extension of the brain), so stretching an arm, for example, will affect the spinal cord between vertebrae C4 and C7/8 (see Figure 3.2 on the next page)

- providing gentle, stroking skin massage (stimulating the A-beta fibers—touch receptors—and the muscle spindles). Massage, as well as hugging, can heal. Frequent hugging and massage are known to produce endorphins and oxytocin. Oxytocin mediates stress, well-being, social interaction, growth, and healing. It lowers blood pressure and heart rate, protects against infection, helps wound healing, and reduces the stress response (see Chapter 4 for more about the healing effects of touch)

- supporting the thoracic spine with sturdy adhesive tape, which helps maintain extension of the thoracic spine, thereby improving general back posture and position of the head, re-educating weak back muscles, and often relieving backache, especially that caused by sitting in front of a computer for long periods

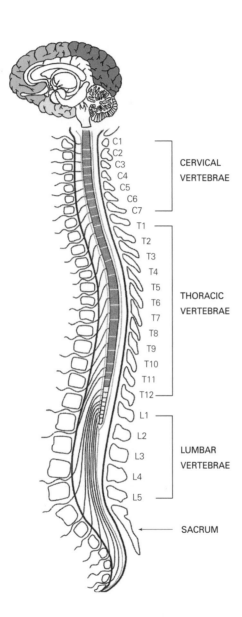

FIGURE 3.2. Regions of the spine

C1
C2
C3
C4
C5
C6
C7

CERVICAL
VERTEBRAE

T1
T2
T3
T4
T5
T6
T7
T8
T9
T10
T11
T12

THORACIC
VERTEBRAE

L1
L2
L3
L4
L5

LUMBAR
VERTEBRAE

SACRUM

Relaxation

Speaking at the Technology Assessment Conference of the National Institutes of Health in 1995, Herbert Benson, who is credited with developing the concept of the "relaxation response," pointed out that leading experts had concluded that relaxation techniques should be incorporated into the treatment of all forms of chronic pain.

Benson defines the relaxation response as "an inducible, physiological state of quietude and the ability to heal and rejuvenate our bodies. The relaxation response is vital to our survival rate in these modern times as it enables us to reduce the anxiety and tension which often inappropriately trigger the 'fight-or-flight' response in us. The 'fight-or-flight' reaction releases cortisol, which if present in large quantities or persistently over time, damages our nervous system, affecting the heart, hormonal system, and metabolism."[19]

As a result of Benson's work on the relaxation response, a U.S. Senate committee in 1999 issued a report that states:

> The Committee recognizes that stress contributes to a host of medical conditions confronted by health-care practitioners, and current pharmaceutical and surgical approaches cannot adequately treat stress-related illnesses. Mind and body approaches, particularly those of the relaxation response and those related to accessing the beliefs of patients, have been used successfully to treat these disorders.[20]

It is impressive that even governments can accept the fact that relaxation techniques are beneficial to health and are an aid in healing many disorders.

Relaxation involves a physical attempt to relax tense muscles and a mental effort to calm the mind. It must be consciously undertaken in order to reach an altered mental state that has been described as "ecstatic, beautiful, totally relaxing, at ease with the world, giving peace of mind, a sense of well-being, and pleasurable."[21]

The following are some tips for achieving relaxation:

◆ Sit or lie comfortably in a quiet place.

◆ Alternately tense and then relax each group of muscles, starting with the feet and moving sequentially to the top of the head, until the whole body feels heavy and relaxed.

◆ During this exercise, try to allow your thoughts to become passive and undisturbed. Focusing on a word, sound, or symbol can help clear the mind.

◆ Remember that the object of the exercise is to shut the mind off from extraneous thoughts in order to achieve mental solitude and peacefulness.

The greatest value of relaxation is that it is our own built-in method for counteracting everyday stresses that produce the flight-or-fight response. It is also an important tool for reducing pain and decreasing muscle spasm and tension.

Distraction

Distraction is a form of therapy that many people spontaneously engage in without realizing they are utilizing another tool that can help them minimize the effects of chronic pain.

Many patients report that they have managed to cope more easily with their pain when they have returned to work or participated in absorbing leisure or business activities. Pain itself damages the nervous system, thus affecting the neural circuitry and chemical configuration. When the mind is distracted from the pain with other thoughts, the patient may become unaware of the pain, even if only for a short period. This respite from pain normalizes the neural circuitry and produces chemicals (endorphins) that are beneficial to healing, which precipitates longer periods of pain relief.

These effects were demonstrated by a study in which eight healthy subjects experienced experimentally induced pain in order to examine the underlying neural systems and mechanisms of pain perception with and without a distracting thought-provoking task. Diminished pain scores from distraction were associated with increased activity in the brain's orbitofrontal region (area for sight) and perigenual cingulated region (deeper limbic system related to emotion and memory). In addition, distraction caused decreased activity in the thalamus (pain-information relay center) and mid-cingulate regions. The insular cortex is interesting because it receives information of sensation from the thalamus, is involved in evaluating the intensity of pain, and interacts with the autonomic nervous system, which we now realize reduces or increases activity of the sympathetic nervous system.[22]

Pain that is ignored or given no value by the logical brain may become less important and may reduce to insignificance. The power of the thought processes in healing and pain relief should never be underestimated.

Distraction may also be achieved through exercise and physical activities, such as Pilates, yoga, tai chi, water aerobics, aerobics, swimming, running, rock climbing, or other forms of absorbing exercise. These activities compel participants to concentrate their attention and energy on the muscles and movements of the various areas of the body to the exclusion of all other thoughts.

The motor cortex of the brain is the region that activates all movements When this system is triggered, it often facilitates pain relief. But movement habits cannot be changed by drugs or surgery (which is why standard pain-management methods are so often only partially or temporarily effective with chronic pain); they can be changed only by new learning, in this case by developing or reactivating neural pathways that enable a person to move voluntarily and freely with an accurate body sense. The process involves learning or relearning muscular control, whatever the clinical method employed. According to the Hanna Somatic Education model, as many as 50 percent of chronic-pain cases are caused by sensory-motor amnesia (SMA). Its most common sign is poor muscular control caused not by damage of muscles or the brain, but by brain conditioning following injury or long-term stress.[23]

The measurement of pain relief requires analysis of movement. Without relieving the pain, movement cannot improve, and without improving movement, there can be no pain relief. It is, therefore, evident that the motor (movement) and sensory (sensation of pain, pleasure, or anything else) regions of the brain have to work together for normal functioning. Recent studies on functional magnetic resonance imaging (fMRI) have demonstrated that a simple injury, such as stubbing the big toe, will activate many areas of the brain, including the motor (movement) regions. A fMRI demonstrates changes in blood flow to motor regions when sensory stimulation (e.g., stubbing the big toe) occurs.

◆ ◆ ◆

I would like to reassure chronic-pain patients that the body does have the ability to heal and rejuvenate itself, given the correct physical and psychological environment. The key is that you need to have the desire and the will to find ways to help yourself that suit your own condition and temperament. You must be persistent enough to continue on the road to healing until success is achieved. Recognize that success may not be complete resolution of the problem, but if your treatment regimen gives you back control and improves your quality of life, you are indeed succeeding!

CHAPTER 4

THE PLACEBO EFFECT AND ALTERNATIVE TREATMENTS

The *placebo* response or effect is the non-specific psycho-physiological therapeutic effect produced by any therapy.[1]

According to the late Patrick Wall, a renowned pain scientist, "If you have a strong enough reason to expect a pain to disappear, it may disappear." The placebo response is valuable because it may, for example, enhance a medication prescribed for pain. If a treatment is accompanied by great expectations, yet has no specific analgesic action, then the decrease in pain is achieved entirely by the placebo response (expectation response).[2]

The placebo effect is healing, is potentially very powerful, and can produce modifications in the central nervous system circuitry, including the autonomic, neuro-endocrine, and neuroimmune systems.[3] It has been demonstrated to improve some conditions by 50 to 90 percent.[4] Herbert Benson refers to the placebo effect as "remembered wellness" that relies heavily on the beliefs of the patient and taps the innate power within the body to heal itself in certain circumstances. Unfortunately, the placebo effect is not a panacea. For instance, no amount of belief in a potion or other treatment will cure a burst appendix; an appendectomy will be needed.

The Mind-Body Connection

We can help ourselves to improve
or we can help ourselves to deteriorate—
the choice is ours!

The placebo effect demonstrates the power of the mind. If possible, it should be harnessed in all treatments. It is the fulfillment of an expectation of a beneficial effect. It is an action that experience has taught may be followed by relief and that depends on a few factors:[5]

- Expectation of the patient
- Belief of the patient
- Trust in the therapist
- The care and respect received from the therapist
- The action of a treatment
- The ritual of treatment

I would like to demonstrate these effects by citing a case history:

FEMALE PATIENT, AGE FIFTY-NINE

Diagnosis: osteoarthritis of the knee. The patient was in the placebo arm of a study that compared transcutaneous electrical nerve stimulation (TENS) APS therapy (modified direct current) with a placebo APS therapy device.[6] Each patient randomly received six treatments. This patient told me that she had achieved wonderful pain relief. She maintained this improvement for an entire year, during which she was able to lead a normal life, including playing tennis, before the pain returned. Although she eventually had to have a knee replacement, a year-long reprieve is well worth the effort, even though the outcome did not change, and demonstrates the tangible power of the placebo effect.

Another study demonstrated that verbal instruction about the treatment will affect the outcome.[7] All patients involved in the study had chest surgery (thoracotamy) followed by buprenorphine injections for pain over the subsequent three days. An infusion of saline was given simultaneously. The members of the first group were not told what was in the infusion, the members of the second group were told that the infusion was either a potent pain killer or a placebo, and the members of the third group were told that the in-fusion was a potent pain killer. Although the analgesic treatment was exactly the same for all three groups, the second group requested less buprenorphine (pain relief) than the first group, and the third group requested less than either the first or second group.

In another study, experimental arm pain was induced in two groups of healthy volunteers.[8] The first group was given an analgesic by injection that was visible to them, and the second group was given an analgesic injection hidden from view by a screen. It was found that the hidden injections produced less pain relief than the visible injections.

Patrick Wall, in his book *Pain: The Science of Suffering*, writes, "*Expectation* of effect is a powerful factor in pain relief and is visible even when medications are used in trials for many other conditions—asthma, cough, diabetes, ulcers, vomiting, multiple sclerosis, and Parkinsonism. Even trials of therapy affecting mood states, such as anxiety, depression, and insomnia, will challenge the investigator's ability to separate the 'true' action from the *suggestion* that the therapy ought to work."[9]

Expectation breeds excitement and anticipation and is compounded by *knowing* that something has been given or done to us to help the pain and that the pain *will* be relieved. Once we "know," the belief system is activated and the body (and brain) starts to work at healing itself. The healing occurs through the nonspecific release of endogenous opioids.[10] We are, therefore, capable of relieving ourselves of pain in certain circumstances.

Beliefs can have a powerful influence on an outcome or effect. This is due to the fact that either something has been proven previously to the individual and the person "knows" through experience that a certain treatment really works, or the person has "seen" a treatment help another individual. An activity and an effect have been established.

For a patient to believe in and have confidence in a therapy, the interaction between therapist and patient should be based on the therapist's having respect for the patient and the patient's having trust in the therapist. When the patient is greeted properly, makes eye contact with the therapist, can express emotions and problems related to the condition in the knowledge that the therapist is caring and listening, senses that he or she is being believed and taken seriously, and feels comfortable in the environment and comfortable about the treatment, efforts at achieving pain relief will likely be more successful.

When something *active* has been done for the patient, he or she begins to relax, stress and anxiety diminish, and the patient knows that the problem is being addressed. All of these factors contribute to the release of the patient's own endogenous pain-relieving and healing mechanisms. The individual's own opioids are preferable to exogenous drugs, because the system releases the necessary and applicable amounts of substances for the particular individual in his or her particular circumstances.

The ritual of treatment is also important and part of the placebo effect. A patient feels more comfortable when he or she knows that he or she is receiving a specific treatment in a particular sequence, for example, laying on of hands, specific exercises, or even a list with advice and/or exercises.[11]

Explanations are another important aspect of the placebo effect. Patients need to have knowledge of the treatment they are about to receive; they must know what the treatment will do, how it will change their condition, and how it has helped others with similar conditions. Patients also need encouragement and frequent reassurance to persist with treatment.

During treatment, it is helpful to demonstrate a change in the pain or movement; if patients see a difference before, during, and after treatment, they will be convinced that the procedure works and that *they chose* the correct treatment for their own condition. The satisfaction of the "customer" is the goal of treatment.

Nocebo is the opposite of placebo and has been called "placebo's evil twin." It is anything that induces a feeling of ill health for no apparent reason. Nocebo takes place through words that undermine confidence or report bad news, such as pronouncing that the patient has a life-threatening disease. The information contained in the contra-indications of a medication also constitutes "something that makes us worse," rather than better.

Too much information can be distressing and damaging to patients. For instance, if a patient reads on the Internet about another person's bad experience with medical interventions for a condition that seems terrifyingly similar to his or her own, they may think, "I had better get to the doctor; otherwise, I may find similar things happening to *me!*" This thought pattern has negative consequences, both physiologically and psychologically, and can undermine a positive response that could have been achieved without this information and expectation.

It has been postulated that a placebo failure may occur because the patient may be unable to produce the requisite amounts of opioids (natural pain relievers), due to changes in or loss of opioid receptors on certain nerve-fiber terminals. Certain patients, for example, have low levels of serotonin in their bodies and thus cannot easily produce their own pain-relieving molecules.

Finally, here is an interesting twist on the power of the mind-body connection: A study was conducted on two groups of rats. One group was fed normal rat food and the other was fed sweets and cookies. A metal plate located under the feeding rats was gradually heated. The rats that were fed normal rat food hopped off the plate when they felt warmth, but the rats that were fed the sweetened food stayed on the plate longer. This indicates that a decision was made to endure possible discomfort for the sake of enjoying a reward.[12]

A similar mechanism probably also occurs in humans. We often decide, whether consciously or unconsciously, to remain in an uncomfortable situation if there is a reward for doing so. I would comment with great respect that this may subconsciously happen with some patients who receive a "reward" (e.g., increased attention from loved ones) for staying in a chronic-pain situation (i.e., they continue to voluntarily suffer the pain in order to receive the pleasurable attention).

Aura Healing

Other forms of healing exist that are not easily understood or accepted because they impart few visible signs of activity and patients may experience inexplicable sensations. One such example is aura healing. The aura is believed to be a band of light energy that is emitted from an individual or an inanimate object. Kirlian photography is thought to capture this energy on film. An aura healer claims the ability to see and manipulate this energy, thus increasing healing in the patient.

The healer may inform the patient that, by working on the aura, healing or improvement will take place in the physical body and the psyche. If the patient feels better and improves both physically and emotionally, this treatment has proven its value to the patient, regardless of whether aura healing can be scientifically proven.

I would like to record a comment made by a patient (male, forty-nine years) who attended an aura healer to treat his depression and uncontrollable tears:

My life used to have huge highs and lows; I now have a calmness about myself and I have so much energy. I am able to train with ease after not being able to do any exercise for five years, as I was always tired. Now when I sleep, it is for an average of six hours, and it's so deep I awake knowing I have slept well. After only a few sessions, I climbed on my bicycle and rode twenty-three kilometers the first time out. During the "treatment," I can feel the energy going through my body and I am able to speak to the healer about my feelings. For the first time in my life, I can love myself. I have changed my way of dressing, eating, hairstyle. I am doing things that I have always dreamed of doing, and it's so easy.

The Power of Prayer

There is a growing body of scientific evidence and acknowledgement by a few in the medical profession that prayer can be effective in medical healing.

In his book *Healing Words,* Dr. Larry Dossey points out that, in some instances, prayer works: "[T]he evidence is simply overwhelming that prayer functions at a distance to change physical processes in a variety of organisms, from bacteria to humans. These data are so impressive that I have come to regard them as the best-kept secrets in medical science."[13]

The following are samples of studies that have been done on the health of people with strong religious beliefs and/or who use prayer frequently:[14]

- In a long-term study of mortality, 5.4 percent of churchgoers died, compared to 17.3 percent of non-churchgoers.

- In a study of disability among the elderly due to illness or injury, lack of religious faith was an even stronger predictor of disability than unhealthy lifestyle.

- A study of high blood pressure found that religious people were 40 percent less likely to have diastolic hypertension than nonreligious people.

- In a study of coronary heart disease, religious men had a 20 percent lower incidence of heart disease than nonreligious men.

- A study of immunity found that nonreligious people had twice as much of a protein that indicates immune weakness (interleukin 6) as did religious people.

- In a study of cancer patients, patients who received a program of spiritual counseling lived approximately twice as long after diagnosis as patients who did not receive this type of counseling.

I believe that prayer for oneself, by oneself, establishes a connection to a higher consciousness, instigates quietude within the mind (contemplative meditation), and empties the mind of emotions. Calming the mind's frenetic activity may stimulate endorphins and anti-inflammatory agents to induce healing. Prayer or meditation facilitates inner-directed action that has no fear or judgement and results in tranquility and the acceptance that pain or disease is a natural part of life.

Quiet contemplation produces a relaxed, tranquil mind through activation of the parasympathetic nervous system, which is controlled by the hypothalamus. As discussed, during parasympathetic activity (general relaxation) we are quiet and calm. Breathing is slowed, as is the heart rate. Blood pressure and body temperature drop. In general, muscle tension decreases. The body regenerates and restores for future activity. The effects of therapeutic thoughts can be demonstrated in a biofeedback laboratory, where experiments to lower blood pressure and other parameters by changing thought processes are conducted.

Stark and Benson developed specific instructions for eliciting the relaxation response. Two factors are especially important:[15]

1. Repetition of a word, sound, phrase, prayer, or muscular activity

2. Passive disregard of everyday thoughts that inevitably come to mind

Prayer or meditative thoughts bring peace and rest to the ever-busy and frantic mind searching anxiously for answers. Patients have a choice to invoke a religious or secular affirmation, according to their belief system. Whatever the choice, it seems that this type of invocation quiets the mind and thus produces a relaxing and healing response.

Touch

Touch is an important aspect of healing; it is one of the most healing modalities available to us. We now understand that the touch receptors (A-beta fibers) access the endogenous opiates that improve relaxation and well-being. Different ways of touching (deeper or lighter pressure) stimulate different fibers and produce different effects on the peripheral nerves, spinal cord, and brain. Touching different areas stimulates circulation, calms muscle spasms, and elicits positive emotions.

A handshake or light touch on the shoulder or hand can help develop a bond of comfort and caring between healer and patient in any discipline of medicine.

Many patients, particularly the elderly, develop chronic "skin hunger," a form of deprivation that may have psychological connotations. When patients become older and lose their spouse or companion, they may become deprived of companionship and touch. This can make them feel miserable, depressed, and uncared for, and can affect their general health and happiness.

Skin hunger is most easily treated by a massage, especially to the back, which can help patients feel "good" and relaxed and can diminish muscle spasm and tension. Programs exist that introduce animals to the elderly, the sick, and the disabled to give them the experience of touching, stroking, and caring.

Hugging is good for you, too! There is an entire field of clinical psychology devoted to the study of hugging.[16] Researchers in the 1970s discovered that hugging induces the release of endorphins, which relieve pain and create feelings of euphoria.

In the book *Touching: The Human Significance of the Skin,* by Ashley Montagu, hugging is shown to boost the immune system. Certain areas of the brain develop in response to tactile stimuli; if a baby does not get hugged enough, part of its brain atrophies and its immune system suffers. Patients, especially babies with AIDS, need holding and caring to assist their immune systems. There are organizations, particularly in South Africa, that provide this type of care for these patients.[17]

As mentioned in the preceding chapter, touch also increases levels of the hormone oxytocin. In addition to conferring the benefits listed in the last chapter, oxytocin (along with the hormone vasopressin) excites neural populations in the brain (in the central amygdala) that regulate the expression of fear, mediate serotonin-induced antidepressant effects (help depression), and reduce pain signals. (As an interesting aside, hypnosis also increases oxytocin levels.)

Magnet Therapy

The validity of magnet therapy has not been tested in double-blind clinical trials, which are the gold standard for determining efficacy. Nevertheless, in my experience, magnet therapy has proven to be a simple, inexpensive, and effective treatment for pain and trauma. In particular, it promotes the healing of fractures. Magnet therapy has a wide range of applications because of its ability to influence the magnetic fields in the body. Our bodies are good conductors of magnetic energy, which makes magnet therapy a regenerative holistic therapy.

The survival and well-being of humans, animals, and plants is dependent on the earth's magnetic field. As part of the U.S. space program, an experiment was performed in which mice were raised in specially prepared metal cages that shielded them from the earth's electromagnetic field. Within a few weeks the animals lost their fur and died. The connective tissue in their skin and internal organs showed signs of uncontrolled growth.[18]

Electric currents are able to magnetize a metal wire, which then develops two distinct poles and attracts iron. Electric current is the movement of ions from the negative to the positive pole; this process is identical to the transmission of an impulse in the nervous system. Every active current in the human body creates a small magnetic field. According to Noel Norris, a small, harmless, direct current is induced in the bloodstream as a result of the blood's exposure to the lines of force of a magnetic field.[19]

Iron is contained in hemoglobin, which transports oxygen from the lungs to the rest of the body. When magnetized, the bonded iron particles in the hemoglobin are attracted to the injured site, improving oxygenation of the area. Water or liquid in the body, when exposed to magnetic fields, reacts by splitting into intermolecular bonds; this assists healing by reactivating the system. The trace element copper supports iron in the blood and helps to defend the body against infection and in the building of red blood cells. It is also involved in the metabolism of pigments and in supporting iron absorption and other metabolic processes.[20]

Many studies by researchers have found that magnets assist with muscle spasm, joint pain, rheumatoid arthritis, and other arthritic conditions.[21] Magnets also improve burn injuries and skin wounds after surgery and have been found to relieve keloid or hypertrophic (enlarged) scars.[22]

Magnets have been shown to improve healing of fractures, particularly when the negative pole is used over or near the fracture site.[23] Another treatment offered for nonunion of fractures (in which a cartilage-like link forms instead of bone) is use of a bone-growth stimulator. This device, worn at night, emits a small, subliminal, direct current while producing a magnetic field around the fracture site.

Many other magnetic-field devices have been developed, such as the Medicur, which was produced in the United Kingdom in the early 1990s. It produces a low-level magnetic field measuring thirty centimeters in diameter. It can be worn in a pocket or over the offending region, and its use generally eases pain.

Magnets have also been used to form a "magnetic trap" over an area of shrapnel embedded in a limb or other body part. In 1997, I talked with a surgeon from Sarajevo who had used a magnetic trap to draw shrapnel to the surface over the course of a few days, whereupon he removed the offending fragment by creating a superficial surgical incision.

The polarity of a magnet is named after its pole-seeking ability. If one side of a magnet is attracted to the north pole of a compass, it is labeled the south-seeking pole of the magnet. If the other side of the magnet is attracted to the south pole of a compass, it is the north-seeking pole of the magnet. A magnet's north-seeking pole has a negative magnetic field, and the south-seeking pole has a positive magnetic field. For this discussion, the north-seeking pole magnet (the negative magnetic field) will be referred to as the north pole, and the south-seeking pole magnet (the positive magnetic field) will be referred to as the south pole.

Magnets can produce different effects on the body based on which polarity is applied. These effects include the following:[24]

North pole:

- Supports biological healing
- Reduces pain and inflammation
- Fights infection
- Produces a negative, direct current (direct current effects)
- Normalizes acid-base balance (it alkalizes tissue)
- Increases cellular oxygen
- Reduces fluid retention

- Encourages restorative sleep
- Constricts blood vessels
- Speeds coagulation and decreases capillary bleeding

South pole:

- Inhibits biological healing
- May increase pain and inflammation
- Accelerates microorganism growth
- Causes positive ionization (positive direct current)
- Causes acid metabolic response
- Decreases cellular oxygen
- Increases intracellular edema
- Stimulates wakefulness
- Expands blood vessels
- Increases red-cell production and softens hard capillaries

The average magnetic intensity of the earth is 0.5 gauss (a measure of magnetic field strength); the magnetic power recommended for treatment is from 600 to 2000 gauss. Biomagnets, which contain a barium-ferrite center with a total diameter of half a centimeter or less, are usually advocated.

Most therapeutic magnets are inexpensive. Certain magnets, when applied to the body surface, emit both polarities; these are called dual magnets. They are generally nonspecific and may be used for soft-tissue injuries. Magnets are commercially available at pharmacies, at medical-product companies, and from some therapists.

The effects of simultaneously placing more than one magnet on the body's surface are not necessarily cumulative; however, the application of many magnets at the same time to an injured area may create an overall positive cumulative effect.

Here are some methods for using magnets therapeutically:

◆ Apply the north pole of the magnet to the skin surface in areas of pain and trauma.

◆ The effectiveness the magnet's positioning may be immediately ascertained by asking the patient to perform a movement that was previously painful. If the movement improves instantly, this is the correct positioning for the magnet. If extra magnets are applied, movement should be reassessed for improvement. If the movement or pain worsens, the magnet(s) should be removed and placed in another area or on the meridian or nerve pathway supplying the painful site.

◆ When using magnets, the same rules apply as for TENS, direct current applications, and acupoints (see Chapters 7, 8, and 9).

◆ Magnets may be left in position on the body and taped with a plaster bandage.

◆ The optimum effect of the magnet is typically apparent within three to five days.

◆ After five days, remove the magnet(s) for two days, then reapply if necessary.

◆ Magnets may be retained during bathing or showering activities.

Magnetic fields are also used to detect disease. The most well-known such use is magnetic resonance imaging (MRI) scanning. New technologies, such as functional MRI (fMRI), assist scientists in analyzing the blood circulation in all areas of the brain involved in different pain states and disease. Additionally, researchers are investigating the subtle properties of biological molecules by using very large magnets in a technology known as nuclear magnetic resonance.

Magnetic field medicine can be sophisticated, but many patients experience improved healing and pain relief from the simple placement of magnets as described above.

Laser Therapy

"Laser" is an acronym for "light amplification by the stimulated emission of radiation." Laser therapy uses a single, specific wavelength with a defined frequency that may be visible or invisible, depending on the wavelength, and is measured in nanometers. Light emanates from the lower frequencies (632.8–750 nm), but not from infrared radiation, which is in the higher frequencies (780–1,300 nm). These lasers are nondestructive and do not cut or damage the skin. However, in some cases they do penetrate the skin to a depth of between one and four millimeters, depending on the frequency of the laser.

Lasers are used for tissue healing and pain control. One of the benefits of laser treatment is that it is subliminal. It causes no sensation, and treatment is of a relatively short duration. Lasers have been used to heal wounds and scars by increasing collagen formation, DNA synthesis, and RNA formation, all of which lead to cell proliferation.[25,26,27]

Laser therapy has been used to treat many musculoskeletal conditions, both acute and chronic, such as rheumatoid arthritis, osteoarthritis, bursitis, and various aspects of back pain, such as nerve inflammation and muscle spasm. It has also been used on trigger points and for neurogenic pain such as trigeminal neuralgia and postherpetic neuralgia. Laser therapy may also be applied to acupuncture points on the body and in the ear. It is a comfortable substitute for acupuncture in children.

The only significant danger from lasers is a risk of damage to the cornea when the beam is applied directly to the eye. The use of specially provided dark glasses is advised for both the therapist and the patient when applying laser treatments.

In my experience, most patients benefit from laser therapy.

Acutouch

The acutouch device was developed in 1994 by Korean industrial engineer Chi Kyung Kim, Ph.D. He initially developed it to help his wife, who had suffered a severe stroke and been given no prospect of recovery by either Western medical doctors or Eastern therapists.

Dr. Kim began to study the principles of natural energy and healing, and he used his engineering knowledge to develop a device that combines a powerful magnetic field, far infrared light rays, and a subliminal negative microcurrent. It is designed in the shape of two pens fixed a specific distance apart. The points that make contact with the skin are gold-tipped (see Figure 4.1).

The two "pens" comprise a hexagonal "hexacromanion" system that channels

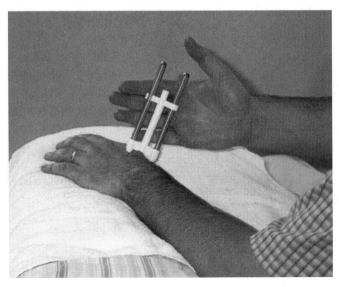

FIGURE 4.1. Acutouch device

and concentrates the energy flow by means of "sympalenses." The healing flow is focused through the tips, which do not penetrate the skin. The far infrared rays help increase the temperature of the deep layers below the skin, widen capillary blood vessels, improve circulation, increase metabolism, and revitalize damaged tissue. The negative ions produced accelerate the delivery of oxygen to the body's tissues, and the magnetic field provides 600 gauss of magnetic energy, which improves circulation, reduces toxins, and delays the aging process of cells. It is known that a tiny electric current in the bloodstream helps eliminate cellular waste in the blood vessels.

Dr. Kim initially designed this apparatus to clear the blockages in blood flow to his wife's brain and to restore her health by balancing her energy according to Eastern principles of medicine. The device channels natural energy into the body at treatment points on the meridians, using the same principles as acupuncture. The resonating lenses draw in and focus natural energy, or chi, together with the far infrared rays, negative ions, and a focused magnetic field.

Kim's wife was treated for many months with the original prototype, opening up the flow of blood and natural energy to her brain. After four months, she recognized him for the first time since her stroke. Two months later, she had regained the power of speech and her memory was restored. By eight months she was walking with the aid of a stick. She now lives a full and healthy life and shows only limited signs of her massive stroke. All the doctors and hospitals that initially attended to Mrs. Kim expressed complete disbelief, but they have now confirmed her recovery.

Since then, acutouch technology has been developed for public use, and many people have used it to treat themselves for chronic ailments and diseases in their own homes. *It cannot be overemphasized that a doctor should be consulted to establish the cause of all ailments and disease before embarking on any treatment.*

Acutouch is usually used in combination with other therapeutic modalities. It can be easily applied at home, although a helper's assistance may be needed if the area requiring treatment is inaccessible to the patient. The basis for treatment is through the acupuncture points and meridians, but it may be used in the same manner or in the same area as the TENS device or any direct current (see Chapters 8 and 9).

When applied on a painful region, such as the spine, a spinous process (which is the protrusion on the center of the back of a vertebral body and the site for the attachment of many spinal muscles), or a medial aspect of the knee joint, acutouch may initially produce uncomfortable sensations. The treatment is maintained until the discomfort disappears. Then another area is selected for treatment. A treatment may require a duration of two minutes in a particular region until the sensitivity diminishes, but thirty to ninety seconds is often sufficient to elicit a healing response.

The value of the acutouch is that it is affordable and easy to use at home, which provides self-control and independence. It is effective for chronic disease or pain. Although the inventor had dramatic results with his wife and many other patients have benefited from the acutouch device, it is not a cure-all for every ailment and has not been tested in double-blinded, randomized clinical trials. It is intended to complement primary treatment for chronic pain. For more information on acutouch and Dr. Kim's device, visit www .acutouch.com.

Homeopathy and Herbal Remedies

Homeopathy is a system of medicine more than two hundred years old that is used on humans and animals and is becoming increasingly popular as a complementary modality. Homeopathy uses infinitesimal doses of substances to influence bodily functions. The idea is similar to that of vaccination, in that low concentrations of a substance are prescribed to the patient to stimulate the body to eliminate that same substance should it appear later in the body at higher concentrations. The problem many Western scientists have with this treatment is that homeopathic remedies are thought to be more potent the more they are diluted, whereas in traditional medicine the opposite is true. There may also be problems combining homeopathic remedies with allopathic (conventional Western) medicine that could cause dangerous side effects.[28]

Little published research exists studying homeopathy's use in managing pain, but there is some evidence for its efficacy, and over the last ten years higher-quality scientific research has been undertaken on its clinical effectiveness. Still, difficulties remain for the scientific study of homeopathy due to the individualized nature of treatment (not everyone is prescribed the same remedy for the same symptoms), the use of combination remedies (in which the medication contains several homeopathic substances), small sample sizes, and the lack of objectively validated outcome measures.[29]

Two major meta-analyses of the clinical effects of homeopathy have been conducted, with both having results that indicate positive effects of homeopathy over placebo. However, the authors found insufficient evidence from these studies that homeopathy is clearly effective for any single clinical condition and called for further rigorous research. No studies have shown effectiveness specifically for pain. Studies of the most popular homeopathic remedy for tissue inflammation, arnica, have failed to show its effectiveness over placebo.[30]

With regard to other herbal remedies, herbalists believe certain herbs and plants are of therapeutic value because of their unique combinations of ingredients. Randomized, controlled trials of herbal remedies have been published, and some positive effects have been reported, but because herbs are not regulated as strictly as drugs are, practitioners (and consumers) must be sure that suppliers adhere to stringent standards of authenticity and preparation.

CHAPTER 5

THE PHYSIOTHERAPEUTIC PERSPECTIVE

P ain that is relieved the moment it presents itself has less opportunity to damage the nervous system than pain that is ignored and that may produce substances that increase pain.

Pain interferes with mobility. Every patient is affected not only by the pain itself but also by the accompanying decrease in muscle strength and tone and by the stffness that limits the range of joint movement. These factors lead to a patient's being disabled in areas both related and unrelated to the pain.

Anxiety, stress, depression, despair, and anger often develop as pain mounts. Relieving these emotions will contribute to a calm mind and improvement in the body's healing capacity. It is therefore obvious that both body and mind need to be assessed in a chronic-pain patient. Then a treatment protocol can be designed to holistically address the patient's condition.

Main Goals of Treatment for the Chronic-Pain Patient

◆ Alleviate and prevent pain

◆ Increase mobility

◆ Decrease anxiety and stress

◆ Improve quality of life

This chapter discusses some of the tools available to the physiotherapist for assessing the chronic-pain patient. It can be useful reading if you are a patient, as you may benefit from understanding the examination procedure and using it to evaluate your own problem. You may arrive at a conclusion that will be helpful in the selection of treatment for your condition.

History Taking

The initial consultation with the patient includes history taking and a physical examination. The history and information concerning presenting symptoms enable the therapist to determine the nature and cause of the problem and to establish a basis for comparison of the progress following treatment. X rays, scans, blood tests, and other information that may relate to the problem should be part of the analysis.

The patient may be invited to write a short synopsis of his or her life story, including the history of the present problem. Professor Birkhan, from the Rambam medical center, in Haifa, Israel, has found that this type of evaluation benefits many patients. The exercise may reveal important information about the physical and emotional sources of the problem, information that is personal and may not necessarily need to be revealed to the therapist or any other person who eventually becomes involved in therapy. Even if details of the patient's life story are shared with no one, the process itself is important, because writing (or painting, in some cases) releases subconscious emotions that the patient does not always recognize or remember. (For more on this topic, see "Narrative Medicine," in Chapter 3.)

Although the assessment process is different for each patient and for each part of the body, the following questionnaire provides examples of typical questions used for pain assessment. Some of these items were taken from the McGill Pain Questionnaire.[1] A few of the categories covered in this sample questionnaire are expanded upon in later sections of the chapter.

Assessment of the Chronic-Pain Patient

The assessment incorporates all relevant details about the patient, including age, occupation, sport/hobby activities, referral information, reason for the referral, and the patient's problem.

I. Subjective analysis

1. History: Present and past

   ◆ A description of how the pain started, how long it has been present, the areas affected, and the activity of the pain.

   ◆ The patient's point of view regarding the pain's cause, his/her future prospects, and his/her current experience.

   ◆ The patient is also invited to tell the therapist about his or her health, body, and life. This narrative information may cause the patient to discover links with previous stress or incidents that may have some bearing on the present situation.

   ◆ The patient's hearing him-/herself communicate, being listened to, and being cared for will improve the patient/therapist relationship and facilitate the activation of descending mechanisms to improve pain relief and the condition itself.

2. A body chart is presented to the patient, who is invited to show/draw on the chart the exact site(s) of the pain.

II. Questions regarding quality of, intensity of, and fluctuations in the pain

◆ Does the pain change with time?

◆ Does the pain feel sharp, cutting, lancinating, hot, burning, scalding, searing, dull, sore, hurting, aching, or heavy?

◆ Which of the following words describe how your pain changes, if at all: continuous, steady, constant, brief, momentary, transient, rhythmic, periodic, intermittent?

Using the above adjectives:

◆ Which word describes your pain right now?

◆ Which word describes it at its worst?

◆ Which word describes it when it is at its least?

◆ Which word describes the worst toothache you have ever had?

◆ Which word describes the worst headache you have ever had?

◆ Which word describes the worst stomachache you have ever had?

◆ Can you sleep at night?

◆ Describe previous surgery or illness(es), or other joint problems.

◆ Describe your general health.

◆ Describe your emotional health.

(Note any unusual descriptions of pain, such as: "the pain is cutting," "like a hot poker," "feels as if I am on the rack," or others. These descriptions may indicate that the nervous system is unduly sensitized and requires medication and/or specific pain treatments to counter the problem.)

How strong is your pain? Use the chart at the bottom of this page to indicate your degree of pain.

◆ Has the pain had any effect on your sense of psychological well-being or your emotional state?

◆ How do you feel about the pain? (See "Emotional Assessment," on the next page.)

◆ What medication(s) are you currently taking?

◆ What treatment helps the condition?

◆ What therapies do you believe may help the condition?

◆ Has anything relevant to your condition/situation not been covered by these questions?

III. Objective examination

Examination of X ray, MRI, or other visual record of the painful area.

Questions follow to indicate functional limitation and disability in specific areas of the body and the ability of the patient to

Mild	Discomforting	Distressing	Horrible	Excruciating
1	2	3	4	5

function at full capacity. Each area has its own functional tests, e.g., how far the knee can be bent, how far the arm can be lifted, how well a fist can be made, etc.

Pain Rating: The Visual Analog Scale (VAS)

Pain intensity is measured on a scale, using a score from 0 to 10 on a line, where 0 indicates no pain and 10 indicates the most severe pain experienced. This is called the visual analog scale (VAS). Ratings for present pain, pain over the past week, or level of pain over the last few months may also be taken.

Place an X on the following line to indicate the level of your present pain:

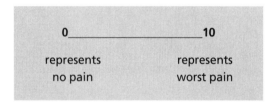

The quality of the pain helps indicate the type of pain experienced. For example, burning, shooting, or throbbing pain may indicate damaged nerves; specific treatment is required to relieve this type of pain.

It is important to analyze the progress made before and after each treatment.

If the pain has not improved by at least 30 percent after three treatments, continuing the current treatment may not be warranted. (An improvement of 30 percent would register 3/10 on the VAS.) The aim of any treatment is to achieve an improvement of at least 50 percent and, hopefully, to reach 80 percent or 100 percent improvement.

The VAS is commonly used, and although not completely accurate in assessing pain levels, it is one of the best assessment tools we have. The reasons for inaccuracies are because pain changes, patients do not always remember well, and any subjective evaluation relates to the way a patient feels at the time of reporting an event, including his or her general state of mind.

It is incumbent upon the therapist to arrive at an accurate assessment of the progress or to demonstrate to the patient the change that has occurred in pain, movements, or condition *after* treatment. Demonstration of a change in movement, swelling, or walking pattern, for instance, develops confidence, trust, and faith in a treatment and its eventual outcome.

Good communication must exist between patient and therapist. The therapist should demonstrate care, listening skills, and belief in the patient. The patient should be able to express him- or herself fully regarding all aspects of the problem, not feel judged, explain how the problem occurred, indicate what he/she feels has caused the problem, and analyze what makes the pain worse or better.

Emotional Assessment

According to Branco Bokun, author of *Humour Therapy,* "[O]ur brain's mental activity is stimulated, ruled, and provided with energy by emotional arousal. Even the slightest difference in emotional arousal can create different conditions within our brain, a difference of mental activity. The brain is also a gland and its glandular activity can be manipulated by thoughts or ideas created by the brain's mental activity."[2]

As has been discussed in previous chapters, emotions govern our mental and physical status. The modern world contains many stressors that affect the responsiveness of the hypothalamic/pituitary/adrenal (HPA) axis, influencing tissue health, recovery, and pain mechanisms. The HPA axis is the interaction of the hypothalamus, pituitary, and adrenal glands. Thoughts that increase our stress levels affect the hypothalamus, which is the master endocrine (hormonal) center for the entire body. It regulates the pituitary, adrenal, thyroid, and sexual glands, among others. The hypothalamus also controls the autonomic nervous system. As described earlier, stress triggers activity within the sympathetic nervous system, which activates secretion of adrenaline and noradrenaline from the pituitary gland, increasing heart rate and blood pressure. Adrenaline increases oxygen consumption in tissues, stimulates the heart, increases cardiac output, and raises the level of energy-providing glucose in the blood, thus increasing the tone of voluntary muscles and creating readiness for action. Noradrenaline reinforces the blood pressure by narrowing the peripheral blood vessels and small arteries. Any increase in activity of the sympathetic system (which is responsible for the fight-or-flight response) reduces activity in the parasympathetic nervous system (which is responsible for the relaxation response), thereby upsetting the body's normal functioning and its homeostasis.

If stress is a constant factor in our lives, the HPA axis becomes the "axis of evil" by triggering the blood pressure and heart rate to remain in a state of readiness for action, the immune system to become overburdened, the hormonal system and metabolic rate to be altered, and the parasympathetic system to become unbalanced. And, of great importance to pain sufferers, stress-caused activation of the HPA increases levels of noradrenaline that may increase or sensitize certain nerve endings. The hypothalamus may also be compromised in its release or control of neurochemicals that improve pain relief. Therefore, we see once again that our thought processes (i.e., our responses to stress) have a powerful effect on our physical body.

The following is a guideline for making an emotional assessment.

Rating the Emotional State

Please describe your mood or general state of mind, based upon the presence or absence of the following emotions/moods/states of mind:

- Tension, anxiety
- Fatigue, inertia
- Depression, dejection
- Confusion, bewilderment
- Anger, hostility
- Vigor, activity
- Overall level of mood disturbance

Describe any other emotions you have, whether positive or negative. The above can be used by patients to mark their own evaluation of their emotional state as desired.

Progress Diary

It is useful for the therapist to encourage the patient to keep a progress diary (see the example on the next page). When a patient is

Day: _____ (e.g., Monday)

How much of each of the following did you do (in minutes or hours)?

	MORNING	NOON	NIGHT
Rest	_____	_____	_____
Sit	_____	_____	_____
Stand	_____	_____	_____
Walk	_____	_____	_____

able to compare notes from the beginning of treatment, any change in physical activities and in pain levels will be evident, thus encouraging and enabling him/her to realize that progress has actually been made. Seeing progress changes perceptions about the condition and improves physiological processes.

Another indication of progress is to compare changes in the following:

♦ Do you have pain at night?

_____

♦ Does it wake you?

_____

♦ How much pain medication or other medication did you take today?

_____

At the end of the initial history taking, patients should be invited to add any information they feel is relevant.

Physical Examination

The physical examination is an objective measure that does not usually relate to the way the patient feels about the condition. It involves measuring movement and observing and evaluating change in the patient. Its goal is to help the therapist decide on the best treatment regimen.

The physical examination may have serious adverse consequences. In certain conditions, forcefully moving joints to detect pain and lack of mobility, or touching a sensitive region, may actually exacerbate the pain. If this is the case, and therefore the therapist cannot touch or manipulate the painful site, examination may include observation or measurement of

♦ active, as opposed to passive, movements

♦ the range and quality of movement

♦ the color and temperature of the area

♦ sweating in the spine, hand, foot, or other areas

♦ hypersensitivity to touch in specific areas

♦ induration, thickening (scar tissue), or tenderness

♦ joint thickness (solid feel) or muscle wasting (indicating weakness)

- the size of the joint or area, in comparison to the other limb/area (e.g., in knee swelling)

- walking distance and speed, if applicable to the patient's condition

If possible, test movements passively. If pain increases abnormally, *stop!*

What Factors Affect Pain?

Many factors can influence pain in an individual patient. The patient needs to be able to help the therapist by giving as much accurate information about the problem as possible. The therapist needs to evaluate all of these factors together to reach a decision about the most appropriate treatment for the condition.

What appears to be the causative factor?

- Is the diagnosis benign?
- Is the condition stable?
- Will continuing treatment and exercise cause damage or increase pain?

What type of problem is it?

- Nerve-related: nerve damage happens when a nerve is pinched or squeezed, or when it is chemically damaged by inflammation; it may also be electrically damaged, as in a neuroma, which can occur in any region of abnormal activity or hyperactivity of a neuron

- Inflammation, stiffness, or damage in a joint

- Muscle problems (e.g., tight and short, inflamed, or weak and lengthened muscles)

- Vascular disturbance due to injury, obstruction, inflammation, or venous ulceration causing skin damage

- Soft-tissue injury, due to damage or contusion (bruising)

- Injury to the skin, producing a wound or scar that may be sensitive, especially after surgery; nerve endings may become irritated and inflamed, producing hypersensitivity in the wound

What is the mechanism of the problem?

It may be one or more of the following:

- Inflammation
- Swelling
- Stiffness
- Circulatory compromise
- Postural
- Stress
- Emotional

Assessment of Nerve Damage

There are two primary types of nerve damage: nerve root compression and "hypersensitive" nerve injury.

Has the pain damaged a nerve pathway, or is it affecting the central nervous system?

- *Nerve root compression:* If a specific nerve has been injured by compression in the low back, it will create leg pain (usually in one leg) in the area supplied by the nerve. It may also produce feelings of pins and needles, numbness, and weakness.

◆ *"Hypersensitive" nerve injury:* If a nerve has recovered from damage only to become sensitized and overresponsive, then some or all of its fibers will increase their responsiveness, both locally and in the spinal cord. In turn, this will influence fibers at higher levels (brain), and the pain may become severe, centralized, and very difficult to relieve.

Where and how does it spread?

◆ See the section on nerve root compression above for a description of the pain pathways in nerve root compression.

◆ The hypersensitive type of nerve injury presents with generalized pain. The pain may spread distally (downward) and create a glove or stocking area on the hand or foot, it may spread proximally (upward) toward the trunk, or it may even develop on the opposite side of the body but in the same region as the original pain (mirror pain, caused when brain circuits become sensitized if the pain is prolonged and/or severe). In some cases, the pain can spread throughout the whole body.

Does it create tenderness?

◆ Nerve root compression may create pain in the spine, buttocks, or legs. Pins and needles and even numbness may be present in the muscles and in the skin supplied by the compressed nerve root. There is usually no local tenderness to the touch in these referred areas.

◆ The hypersensitive type of nerve injury may cause parts of the body, typically limbs, to become very sensitive to touch. The patient may desire to hold the limb very still, for fear of anything touching it, or may avoid performing any movement that could increase the pain. This tenderness can spread into the whole limb, a condition referred to as complex regional pain syndrome (CRPS). In CRPS, a small injury, such as a blow to the big toe, may create disturbance in the whole limb because the central nervous system has become involved.

Has it affected the tissues in the area?

◆ In nerve root compression, the local tissues in the limb will not be damaged.

◆ In hypersensitive nerve injury, the tissues from the skin all the way to the bone may be damaged if the original condition was not treated as soon as possible. The tissues may also become severely irritated, due to increased pain caused by examination or treatment, or by forcing movements through the pain (conventional physiotherapy).

Does the condition increase responses to pain?

◆ Nerve root compression leads to pressure on the nerve in the spinal cord and facet joints, but it does not usually create increased responses to pain.

◆ The hypersensitive type of nerve injury may become increasingly responsive to noninjurious stimulation. It may also become unstable, with pain returning easily, even if relieved. The condition may recur if not properly treated and dissipated within the specific region.

Has it produced dysfunction in the musculoskeletal and nervous systems?

◆ Nerve root compression may cause the nerve to become damaged in the spinal cord, possibly leading to weakness. The condition may resolve eventually, or it may require traction or surgery to release the trapped nerve. Surgery is recommended in very few cases.

◆ Hypersensitive nerve injury could cause the patient to lose the use of the joint or limb. Therefore, the best advice is to use the limb as much as possible.

What suffering has it caused?

Patients who are depressed, anxious, sleepless, angry, and emotional because of their pain are suffering because their quality of life has been affected, they experience loss of control over their lives, and they cannot see any relief becoming available in the future (they anticipate never-ending pain).

Appropriate Treatments for Specific Conditions

Here is a quick summary of treatments often employed by physiotherapists. The list also includes modalities that complement physiotherapy well and are often provided by other practitioners (e.g., acupuncture).

◆ A stiff joint requires mobilization and

exercise that restore the joint to as normal a range of movement and function as possible.

◆ Nerve compression is usually relieved by a specific treatment or a combination of treatments—for example, mobilization, traction, acupuncture, electric currents, wearing a brace, and/or exercise.

◆ Specific electric currents, acupuncture, skin applications, and medication for pain and swelling reduce inflammation.

◆ Electric currents, acupuncture, magnets, medication, and exercise improve circulation to increase the blood supply.

◆ Exercise and taping can correct poor posture that causes pain, stiffness, and weak and elongated muscles. It also releases the antagonistic muscles that have tightened and shortened.

◆ If pain is the main component, then blocking the pain with acupuncture and selected electric currents will also improve other symptoms.

◆ If stress affects the pain, then relieving stress with electric currents, acupuncture, exercise, visualization, breathing, and meditation will help to solve the problem.

◆ ◆ ◆

It is important for the therapist to remember that many patients need both emotional and physical support to heal their stress, anxiety, and pain.

CHAPTER 6

THE PAIN PATHWAYS

The nervous system consists of a network of nerves that mobilize the muscles, interact with the autonomic nervous system and blood vessels, relay information from the periphery to the brain, and activate the brain. Sensory information on pain is relayed by specific nerve endings: the pain receptors (nociceptors). Nociceptors are found in the skin, joints, muscles, and viscera (internal organs).

Sensation usually involves the largest organ of the body, the skin. The skin relays information from the periphery to the spinal cord and on to the brain. The peripheral nervous system consists of sensory, motor, and autonomic nerves.

The brain's processing of information from the periphery is affected by memory and by whatever emotions we are experiencing at the time. The psychological response is followed by a complex physiological reaction that either permits the sensation to continue, or removes the body from the noxious or harmful experience. Sensations are also relayed from the internal environment by nerve endings (visceral nerves) that travel along different pathways and are unavailable to manipulation or touch.

As you can see, various bodily systems are activated when any experience, mental or physical, occurs that involves our periphery and our proximity. Information is relayed by specific pathways in a manner similar to trains that operate on the outskirts of a city. The trains run on designated tracks toward the city, reach the suburbs near the city (substations), and then continue until they reach the main central station within the city.

Types and Functions of Nerve Fibers

Different kinds of nerve fibers relay different types of information, such as touch, warmth, cold, and pain. The pain receptors, or nociceptors, are the neuron's afferent (incoming) fibers. The fibers that relay information from a noxious or painful input consist of two types: C fibers and A-delta fibers. The C fibers are thin, conduct slowly (one meter per second), and have no fatty sheath covering them (i.e., they are unmyelinated). They are sensitive to mechanical stimulation, temperature, and irritating neurochemicals, and they relay information on temperature, pressure, and pain. C fibers connect with the autonomic nervous system.

A-delta fibers are slightly thicker, thinly myelinated, faster conducting (fifteen meters per second), and also relay information on temperature and pressure.

A-beta fibers are a third type of nerve fiber. They are responsible for pain inhibition. We are constantly stimulating A-beta fibers without even realizing it. They are thicker, fully myelinated, activated by touch and pressure, and much faster conducting (fifty meters per second) than the other fibers. This means that the information from touch reaches our brain *before* information on pain. When we notice a sensation, whether uncomfortable or not, we may place a hand on the area. If it is painful, we may press, rub, hit, or even vibrate the region. When we instinctively stimulate these A-beta fibers, we release pain-relieving substances in the area of the pain as well as in the spinal cord and brain. We thereby disturb or interrupt the pain pathways via another pathway (touch) that reaches the brain first. This mechanism blocks the pain.

The A-beta nerve fibers are not normally hypersensitive. If, however, sensitization occurs in the nervous system, they may become painful and overly sensitive when stimulated by pressure or touch.

Another method of easing pain is to change the temperature. Activating the thermoreceptors (nerve fibers that respond to heating, i.e., the C and A-delta fibers) may thereby also decrease pain. Some patients respond to warmth and others to cold. We spontaneously use the modality or activity that makes us feel more comfortable or eases the pain. We may have to try different temperatures or pressures, but, in any case, "what feels good often produces pain relief." Activities that utilize temperature and touch may be used in our coping strategies.

Other nerves that act even faster than the A-beta (touch) fibers are the A-alpha fibers. They conduct at one hundred meters per second and are situated in muscle spindles in the skeletal muscles. When movement or muscular activity occurs, it may interfere with the pain pathways. This is why it's important to continue moving and to maintain activity as another pain-blocking mechanism.

As information travels along these nerve fibers toward the spine, it first reaches a small substation, the dorsal root ganglion (collection of nerve fibers), then proceeds into the posterior (rear) nerve root as it enters the posterior aspect of the spinal cord. In the spinal cord, these fibers penetrate different layers of the spinal cord (major substation) where they may connect to other fibers in this region, or to the nerves that connect with the periphery (outside of the body), or to the sympathetic ganglia that are part of the chain of the autonomic nervous system that runs in front of the thoracic spine. These ganglia are made up of a bundle of nerve tissue that receives incoming (from the spinal cord) and outgoing (to the target tissue) nerve fibers.

The above information has been simplified. Complex interactions are constantly taking place, as described in the first chapter. It is important to examine all areas of the nervous system that offer the opportunity to disrupt the pain pathways in order to demonstrate that patients have the ability to block pain and to produce their own natural pain relievers and anti-inflammatories by using electrical devices or other activities that stimulate different systems.

After the Injury

Once an injury, muscle spasm, or other damage occurs (for example, a sprained back muscle), a local reaction takes place that produces inflammation (via histamine, mast cells, neutrophils, and prostaglandins); it is followed by an immune response and the release of endogenous (natural) endorphins (pain relievers) that help to reduce both the inflammation and pain. The injury itself produces electrical information that is transmitted through neurons to the spinal cord and the autonomic nervous system, and then extends to the sensory and motor cortex in the brain.

As the information passes through these areas, many different chemical substances are produced, such as inflammatory mediators (bradykinin, prostaglandins, leukotrienes, serotonin, histamine, substance P, protons, thromboxanes, platelet-activating factor, free radicals, cytokines, adenosine and adenosine phosphates), depending on the degree of disturbance in the nervous system. At the same

time, endorphins (beta-endorphins, dynorphins, enkephalins) and monoamines (melatonin, serotonin, noradrenaline) are released at different levels of the nervous system to relieve pain. The effect of this reaction may also release substances in the autonomic (thoracic ganglia) nervous system. These substances, such as adrenaline and noradrenaline, initially help the condition, but if the response is prolonged due to ongoing relentless pain, sensitization of nerve endings and of the whole nervous system occurs, resulting in adverse health consequences.

Once received within the sensory cortex of the brain, all information passes through a multimodal region that involves, among other structures, the hypothalamus and pituitary, with extensive processing occurring before the information reaches the motor cortex. The hypothalamus is responsible for hormonal, autonomic, and neurochemical activities that, as previously mentioned, assist the body in maintaining homeostasis. There are also nuclei in the hypothalamus that are responsible for controlling mental and physical states such as rage, satiety and hunger, body temperature, urination, and sexual emotions. The pituitary is responsible for hormonal release that affects all the peripheral endocrine organs.

Ascending or incoming information on pain may be affected, controlled, or blocked by specific stimulation at the level of the periphery, spinal cord, autonomic nervous system (sympathetic), midbrain, medulla, thalamus, or sensory cortex. This stimulation may occur by means of chemical mediators (medication), electric currents, acupuncture, temperature changes, or other interventions.

Depending on the memory and emotions released at the time of injury, reactions occurring in the hypothalamus, pituitary, hormonal, and autonomic regions of the brain result in the release of neurochemicals that will either increase or diminish the pain experience. An important pathway descends through each region: from the higher centers in the brain through the midbrain, medulla, spinal cord, and sympathetic ganglia to the injury site. It is called the descending pathway, and it can be activated by "increasing pain" at a distal site to the injury, or at the injury itself. This increase in pain is called counter-irritation and may be activated by applying a painful yet controlled stimulus to the area. This is the philosophy behind such modalities as plum-blossom needling, periosteal pecking, or certain electric currents. Certain medications that burn or irritate may also activate these pathways. The descending mechanism is also activated by breathing exercises, relaxation, visualization, meditation, and the release of endorphins from whatever activities may produce these substances (e.g., exercise).

Figure 6.1 on the next page shows a simplified graphic of the ascending and descending pathways, and of how different types of stimulation can block pain.

It should be clear from this discussion that any sensory stimulus, such as pain, is affected by complex processes and thus produces effects that may be difficult to resolve.

Neural Damage

Chronic-pain patients potentially face many difficulties when they sustain damage to the neural system.

In the periphery, prolonged trauma associated with tissue damage produces stimulation of the traumatized ends of the afferent nerve fibers, which as a result may continually send impulses either into the same damaged tissue or to all the relay stations in the central nervous system. This is similar to a broken record; it gets stuck in the same place, or on the same message. At the same time, a sensitizing "soup" of chemicals collects around the area, leading to overexcitable sensory and sympathetic nerves and producing unpleasant sensations such as burning, tingling, painful numbness, shooting, sharp pains, constant aching, deep pain, intolerance to touch, and painful movement of joints. This disturbance may affect the skin, soft tissue, muscles, viscera (internal organs), and even bone.

The disturbance in all these nerve endings is similar to a radio that is not tuned in properly, resulting in a barrage of noise instead of music. It can alter nerve fibers near and far, with reception being affected all the way to the brain. The receptor sites become damaged so that they no longer respond to normal electrical stimulation or chemical modulation. Some areas become depleted of certain substances, such as serotonin, resulting in increased pain and autonomic and sleep disturbances, such as in fibromyalgia. Imbalance may also occur in the hypothalamus and in the autonomic or hormonal systems. Patients with diabetes, for example, could develop diabetic neuralgias. Noradrenaline, which is necessary for the reflex control of blood vessels, may be present in below-normal quantities and may influence complex regional pain syndromes.

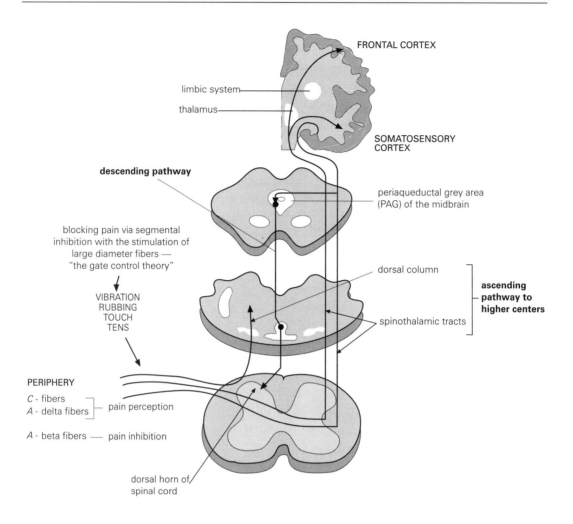

FIGURE 6.1. Blocking the pain leads to pain modulation

The changes in the nervous system mentioned above may lead to increased activity of the neurons in the injured area itself and/or in other areas of the nervous system, which leads to increased pain. Like most cells, neurons are continuously dividing and being replaced, resulting in changes to the system's electrical circuitry. Previous damage to neurons is contained in the cell memory, and this continuance in the new cells will af-fect the DNA; the new neurons may retain the memory of the old neurons and pain may be "remembered" and therefore perpetu-ated within the coded information in the DNA of new neurons.

Changes may also occur in the neuronal cells themselves—both those in the local tis-sue as well as those in the spinal cord and brain—leading to increased responsiveness to pain stimulation. The changes in responsiveness by the neuronal cells are due to the release of certain substances that in turn cause changes in the cell walls, producing a different cell metabolism and increasing the electric excitability of the cell. Nitric oxide may be produced in the circumstances mentioned above; it is now known that nitric oxide is implicated in chronic-pain states, acting as a positive feedback in the maintenance of pain. Its presence may lead to cell death, with long-term alterations in the responsiveness of the cells.

◆ ◆ ◆

Again, the complexity of all these changes indicates how difficult it can be to help the chronic-pain patient. Therapists and patients should adopt a trial-and-error approach to exploring different applications. Once a successful pain-blocking treatment, medication, or device is found, the patient must take responsibility for helping him- or herself by using it consistently. Such self-treatment can ease the financial burden that is often placed upon chronic-pain patients, and it may also reduce the need for medical consultations as well as unnecessary investigations and procedures.

CHAPTER 7

What Is Acupuncture and How Does It Relieve Pain?

Acupuncture—the practice in which very thin needles are inserted into the skin at specific sites—is a treatment that originated in China and has been performed there for thousands of years. Knowledge of this healing art was introduced to the Western world in the sixteenth century. In addition, the emigration of many Chinese acupuncturists over the centuries has helped disseminate the recognition of acupuncture as a healing treatment worldwide. The practice remained largely unknown outside of China, however, until the 1950s, when the first reports of surgery under acupuncture anesthesia appeared. The revolutionary government in China actively encouraged the rebirth of acupuncture. Interest gradually filtered to the West and Europe, especially after Nixon's visit to China in the 1970s, when people began to realize that acupuncture is a suc-cessful treatment for many conditions, including chronic pain.

Many patients throughout the world who have experienced acupuncture vouch for its effectiveness. Their anecdotal support, together with the emergence of scientific evidence over the last twenty years from major universities in both China and the United States, has caused acupuncture to become accepted not only by the public but also by Western medical practitioners, the U.S. government, and medical funding organizations in Europe.

Energy in the Body

Acupuncture sites, or points, as they are known, are situated on pathways in which bioelectric energy, known as qi (pronounced "chee," and sometimes spelled *chi*), is propagated. These pathways are called meridians or channels. It is interesting to note that most pain impulses travel along the same pathways as those of traditional qi circulation. Special points also exist that are not on the meridians but that may be situated in or near a painful area or joint, or that have specific general effects on the body when needled.

It is difficult for Westerners to accept the fact that energy exists in the body and that healing takes place when energy points are stimulated. The difficulty lies in the fact that medical science teaches that we must measure physical changes in order to analyze disease. Yet these energy pathways cannot be seen. When a person dies, the acupuncture points cannot be viewed anatomically, either with a microscope or with the naked eye. On the living body, however, they can be detected by electrical measurement.

Acupuncture points on the living body have a lowered electrical resistance due to the rich supply of blood vessels and nerve endings that are found under the skin in these regions. Researchers have indicated that 309 acupoints lie on or near the nerves and that 286 acupoints are situated next to major blood vessels, which are surrounded by small nerve bundles. The increased fluid in the region produces a reduced resistance when detected electronically by a "point finder." A point finder is a small device that was originally derived from the work in the 1940s and '50s of J.E. Niboyet, who used a galvanometer to detect electrical conductance on acupuncture points. When it is placed on a true acupuncture point, it emits a beep to indicate that the resistance has changed. Acupuncture points have a conductance between 5 and 50 kilo-ohms, whereas nonacupuncture points have a conductance between 0.5 and 3 mega-ohms.[1,2]

The low resistance of acupuncture points is yet another confirmation of the existence of electricity within the body. Actually, the "energy" within the body that can be elicited by acupuncture lies in the "power of the nerve" (propagation of energy along the channel, or an electric charge stimulated in the nerve) in the area being treated.[3] Nerve tissue transmits information along its fibers by means of an electric charge; this information is relayed to larger nerve fibers, to the spinal cord, and ultimately to the brain. An electric charge along a nerve fiber is the energy "currency" of the nervous system.

The meridians pass over the skin, mostly in a longitudinal direction, and connect via internal channels to the internal organs. As explained above, these internal channels are not anatomically visible, but they may be identified by the energy they propagate or by the influence they have on different bodily systems. Ancient doctors discovered that when they drew lines to connect effective needling points with the parts of the body that were most affected by the needling, they were able to make a visible representation of a channel that connected all the points together; in modern times these acupuncture channels became the "meridians."

Insertion of needles into a point on a meridian may influence either a local region or another, remote area. The needles influence the health of the body and create balance in all the systems, including the autonomic, metabolic, hormonal, and nervous systems. Acupuncture tends to balance the physiological function of the body, rather than stimulating or reducing it, thereby helping to maintain homeostasis.

Personal Observations

Acupuncture has made a deep impression on me. When I first started studying acupuncture in the late 1980s, I was asked to insert needles into a patient's ear to treat her cervical spondylosis (neck osteoarthritis) and shoulder pain. To my amazement, even my inadequate skill as a novice at inserting and finding the relevant points in the ear representing the neck, shoulder, and Shen Men (a major calming point) produced greatly improved movements and pain relief in the patient. She had been receiving physiotherapy at the Johannesburg General Hospital for six months prior to our meeting, and had enjoyed little if any sustained improvement.

Over the years, as I treated many patients with acupuncture, I observed that results were obtained much more rapidly than with conventional physiotherapy and with even greater success when acupuncture was combined with physiotherapy. I noticed that patients often demonstrated changes in their demeanor. They were

- relaxed during treatment and often fell asleep
- emotional (some even shed a tear)
- more communicative, sharing information about themselves that seemed to stem from emotional problems, or from events that had long been forgotten

I always noticed that when patients returned for the next treatment, especially after an "emotional" response, they were better! When I began using acupuncture on chronic-pain patients, I always noticed improvements in their mobility. When pain was relieved, function also improved.

So How Does Acupuncture Really Work?

This is the question many patients and students of acupuncture want to have answered.[4]

Acupuncture needles create tiny lesions in the skin that take two to five days to heal. For this reason the effects of treatment are not always immediately visible. The needles may be inserted either in local tender points or in designated points along meridians near the pain site. As a result, the body reacts by mobilizing the anti-inflammatory agents of the immune system and stimulating the release of endorphins (the body's natural pain relievers).

Acupuncture points exist in collaboration with sensory nerves or with tissues supplied by sensory nerves. Sensory nerves transmit information from the periphery to the spinal cord to activate spinal neurons. Needling the skin stimulates certain fibers in the sensory nerves that send impulses toward the spinal cord and brain along various pathways. Specifically, it stimulates the A-delta, A-beta, and C fibers, which, as you may remember from the preceding chapter, are involved in pain pathways. Depending on the type, size, and thickness of the nerve fibers, different pathways are activated to target the release of endorphins (polypeptides that reduce pain sensitivity) or neurotransmitters (natural pain relievers), such as enkephalin, dynorphin, and serotonin, in different areas of the spinal cord and brain.

Enkephalin and dynorphin inhibit incoming pain messages to the spinal neuron. The spinal neuron stimulates spinal-thalamic pathways that extend to the sensory cortex of the brain; thus, endogenous pain relievers are released both locally and throughout the nervous system. This occurs through interaction between the various brain centers. The hypothalamus and pituitary release beta-endorphin into the blood and cerebral spinal fluid, promoting physiological pain relief and homeostasis. (In addition to mechanisms that promote tissue healing, as mentioned, acupuncture also influences the immune, cardiovascular, and respiratory systems.) The hypothalamus, by secreting adrenocorticotrophic-stimulating hormone, activates the adrenal glands to modify pain and the immune reaction.

The brainstem is the major site of production of the neurochemicals acetylcholine and noradrenaline, among others. Acetylcholine is released by neurons that pass to the spinal cord, by all of the parasympathetic neurons, and by some sympathetic neurons. Noradrenaline (also called norepinephrine), a product of adrenaline that stimulates the sympathetic nervous system and also modulates pain in certain areas and situations, is released by most sympathetic neurons. It has been observed that when pain thresholds are elevated (i.e., when the patient feels less pain), levels of norepinephrine are reduced in the cortex, hypothalamus, brainstem, spinal cord, and striate body, thus having an effect opposite that of endorphins, which are elevated in these areas. The autonomic nervous system is activated by stress, and it may be postulated that when noradrenaline levels are elevated (through stress), they may reduce pain thresholds, causing the patient to feel increased pain.

This mechanism indicates that the body has its own resources to heal itself and produce pain relief, depending on the health status and the self-healing capacity of the individual and the potential for healing of various symptoms.

Another aspect of acupuncture healing is the stimulation of homeostatic points. These are points that have been discovered to have nonspecific effects on the body, for example for nausea or relaxation. Certain points normalize or balance activities of the sympathetic system (when it is overactive) or parasympathetic system (when it is underactive) to restore optimal homeostasis. The nonspecificity of these points facilitates treatment for many different conditions. Other homeostatic points balance the hormonal, metabolic, and nervous systems.

If acupuncture is applied to the skin above the spine (paraspinal) to influence the specific nerve roots that supply the area of pain, then transmission of pain signals may be reduced or relieved, and healing (for muscle pain, spasm, poor circulation, and inflammation) takes place in the affected region.

Insertion of the metal acupuncture needle creates a short circuit across the skin "battery," creating a microcurrent that stimulates healing. Existence of this current indicates that the body requires electrical current to stimulate healing in diseased or damaged areas that suffer aberrant nerve conduction or poor circulation. Mechanical stimulation by the needle itself deforms (stretches) the connective collagen and elastic fibers in the tissues, which in turn sends signals for tissue healing to nerve centers, small and large.

Another aspect of needle insertion is the effect of the "needle injury." The needle creates a micro-injury in the tissue, and the body responds with an overwhelming reaction of the local defense or immune mechanism. The effect of this response is to repair not only the micro-injury but also the surrounding area of injury or disease. The needle also initiates a potential action or electrical charge in the peripheral nerve (i.e., the limb) or in the spinal segmental nerve (the nerve in the spine that supplies the limb) that it stimulates. This triggers a complex series of biochemical effects—for example, release of opiates (natural pain relievers) and anti-inflammatory substances—as a result of the signals received in the whole nervous system, including the brain.

Acupuncture is extremely effective in treating the musculoskeletal system since the muscles, tendons, ligaments, and bones lie under the skin along the meridians. When muscles are in spasm, inserting a needle into the tight musculature will release the spasm by initially "grabbing" the tight tissue and then relaxing it. A "twitch response" may be noted. When the muscle is compared before and after needle insertion, the muscle feels more relaxed to the therapist, and the patient admits that the previous tenderness has disappeared, usually much to his or her surprise!

Other experts summarize the significant pain-relieving effects of acupuncture as follows:[5]

- It activates the serotonergic system (i.e., the serotonin-release system) in the brain and spinal cord.

- It stimulates the synthesis and release of norepinephrine in different areas of the central nervous system, with a depletion of the substance occurring simultaneously in other tissues. In some areas, such as the brain, norepinephrine is antagonistic to acupuncture analgesia (cancels out the effects of the pain relief), and in other areas, such as the spinal cord, norepinephrine facilitates acupuncture analgesia (AA).

- Enkephalin is mediated by AA in the brain and spinal cord.

- Beta-endorphin is mediated by AA in the brain, but not in the spinal cord.

- Acupuncture is capable of releasing beta-endorphin in the brain, and dynorphin and enkephalin in the spinal cord. (Beta-endorphin, dynorphin, and enkephalin are all endorphins, i.e., polypeptides that reduce pain sensitivity.)

- The frequency (see below) of acupuncture stimulation has been found to stimulate different substances. Therefore, different frequencies will produce different substances in different areas of the nervous system.

In addition:[6]

- Acupuncture excites receptors or nerve fibers in the stimulated tissue that are also activated by strong muscle contractions; the effects are similar to those obtained by protracted exercise.

- Low-frequency electroacupuncture (between 1 and 4 hertz, or Hz) may be effective in treating most conditions, especially those involving inflammatory, injury-related, circulatory, or neuropathic pain. High-frequency electroacupuncture (between 100 and 200 Hz) may ease pain in muscles, especially back muscles, where relaxation is required. (Electroacupuncture involves stimulation of acupuncture points by passing an electrical current through the acupuncture needles. For more on this topic, see Chapter 8.)

◆ Acupuncture may be inefficient in certain chronic-pain patients with high generalized anxiety or pain all over the body (central pain emanating from sensitized brain receptors), possibly due to increased levels of cholecystokinin (an opioid antagonist), other substances, or central (brain and spinal cord) sensitization. This suggests that patients are more likely to respond to acupuncture when they are not stressed or anxious, and it would imply that treatment will benefit from destressing the patient by addressing his or her worries, concerns, and goals and by treating specific acupuncture points that relax and reduce stress before treating the actual condition (see below).

As this section has shown, acupuncture triggers the release of many endogenous substances that relieve pain. Different areas of the brain have specific influences on the autonomic, metabolic, neurohormonal, and nervous systems, all of which can be affected by acupuncture. Different endogenous substances influence different types of pain control, and they influence healing in different areas—in the periphery (area of the injury), spinal, and supraspinal (central nervous system) regions. (For a discussion of acupuncture protocols to treat various conditions, see Appendix A.)

Acupuncture Studies

D. Meyer performed an experiment in which the pain-relieving effect induced by acupuncture in one animal could be transferred to another by transfusion of the cerebrospinal fluid. This means that the body's pain-relieving substances—the endogenous opioids—are produced in the brain and that they can be elicited by acupuncture.[7]

Acupuncture is not a form of hypnosis or a placebo. On the contrary, it has been observed that people who receive acupuncture and do not believe that it will help are just as likely to respond as people who have faith in the treatment. One of the best arguments supporting acupuncture's effectiveness is its successful use in the treatment of many diseases in animals.

Many studies in both China and the West have demonstrated that acupuncture achieves its effect through physical means, using the brain's own biochemistry.[8]

Important studies were presented in June 2005 at the Second International Medical Congress on Acupuncture, in Barcelona. Randomized, controlled trials had been conducted in an extensive acupuncture research initiative sponsored by the German health-insurance company Modellvorhaben der Techniker Krankenkasse.[9] Acupuncture reduced migraine headaches in 302 patients. Pain, function, and physical quality of life were improved in 294 patients with osteoarthritis. Marked improvement in pain intensity and back function was noted in 298 sufferers of chronic low-back pain.

Acupuncture Helps You Move

Acupuncture often has profound and immediate effects on movement. Acupuncture points on the scalp have a close relationship with the sensory and motor areas of the brain and are often used to assist with improving a joint's range of motion. After insertion of a needle into the scalp, the patient is often able to move the joint more freely and with reduced pain. Much to the disbelief of the patient, suddenly an immovable joint becomes free!

Once again, the relationship between movement and pain relief is established. When a patient who had a stiff joint becomes able to move more freely after acupuncture, I recognize that pain was the inhibiting factor in his or her problem. If increased mobility does not occur, I know that the joint itself has an inherent blockage and requires mobilization and anti-inflammatory and circulatory relief by means of acupuncture and other modalities.

A similar effect is observed by needling points in the ear that influence the joints. The ear is a complex system that represents the whole body. In fact, it looks like an upside-down fetus. Many acupuncturists focus only on the study of the ear. The ear can be used to treat every condition known to man, including asthma, addictions, weight gain, stress, and skin disorders, to name a few. Other microsystems in the body, such as the face, long bones, hands, feet, and even the scapula, are said to have acupuncture points representing the whole body. These systems are called ECIWO, short for "embryo containing the information of the whole organ-

ism," and they offer more evidence that the human body has access to many different healing processes within itself.[10]

♦ Acupuncture, due to its effect on movement, enhances rehabilitation.

♦ Acupuncture can enhance recovery in peripheral (outer) nerve injury, neuropathic disease (sensitized nerve endings), and muscles that have sustained partial nerve damage.

Acupuncture and the Emotions

Laughter keeps you young;
anger makes you old.

— Chinese proverb[11]

Chinese medicine makes no distinction between treatment of the body and of the mind; it is essential to treat both simultaneously. The ancients realized that happiness and relaxation had profound effects on the body's internal organs. In the philosophy of Chinese medicine, disease cannot manifest itself when the body and mind function well. Traditional Chinese acupuncture treats sadness, lack of laughter, over-laughter, depression, anger, worry, and many other emotions by using specific points that impact the internal organs and improve general health.

Scientists are now beginning to analyze anger as a major "disease enhancer." I, too, believe that certain types of emotions and thoughts impact our present and future health. Accordingly, I would like to offer the following recommendations:

- Do not harbor negative emotions against yourself or others.

- Do not hold on to your anger.

- Be willing to forgive.

- Do not worry constantly.

- Do not internalize your feelings. Learn to release emotions and to express yourself.

- Be honest with yourself.

- Foster a belief system that sustains you.

- Think good and loving thoughts.

- Smile and laugh as often as possible.

A patient who has pain is usually negative, sad, distressed, worried/anxious, angry, unforgiving, and depressed. Treatment, such as acupuncture, that relieves these challenging emotions will enhance physical healing and pain relief.

Acupuncture for Stress Reduction and Relaxation

Acupuncture treatment focused on points for stress reduction and relaxation is recommended for many patients who are stressed and anxious about their condition and their pain. However, these patients may even be fearful of "having needles stuck into them." Recall from earlier chapters how certain emotional states can reduce the availability of endorphins and anti-inflammatory substances. These effects can limit the positive results of acupuncture. For these reasons, it would benefit pain patients to engage in some form of stress reduction before any other treatment is given.

I have found that allowing time to communicate with the patient and then treating specific relaxation and anti-anxiolytic points (before actually treating the condition) often have a positive effect. I am then able to concentrate the treatment on pain relief and mobility because the "scene" has already been set for relief and relaxation, and the patient is now prepared to get well.

The following are the acupuncture points for stress reduction and relaxation (see Figure 7.1 on the next page). It is not in the ambit of this book to provide instructions for locating these points, but many other books are dedicated to this subject:

- Du 20—scalp (Du meridian point 20)

- EP 1—between the eyebrows (Extra point 1)

- Ren 17 (Ren meridian point 17)

- Li 4 (Large intestine meridian point 4)

- H 7 (Heart meridian point 7)

- Sp 6 (Spleen meridian point 6)

- Liv 3 (Liver meridian point 3)

This combination of points has the following effects:

- Relaxation, even sleepiness

- Deepened breathing, often initiated by a deep sigh

- Release of emotions such as sadness (a tear may fall)

- Pain relief (Li 4 is the major pain-relieving point for all types of pain, including cancer pain)

- Anxiety relief (calms the mind)

- A decrease in depression, a lift in spirits (patients may start to smile or become more communicative)

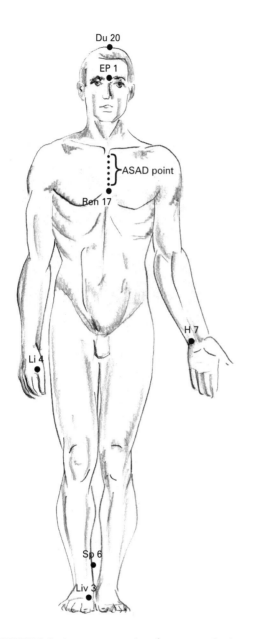

FIGURE 7.1. Acupuncture points for stress reduction and relaxation, as well as for anxiety, nausea, and depression during chemotherapy (ASAD point)

It is interesting to note that the combination of points Li 4 and Liv 3 is also used in the treatment of depression. This is significant, as patients with pain appear to produce the same chemical substances as those with depression. Recent trends in pharmacology advocate administering antidepressive medication in relatively low doses to relieve pain. Another interesting fact is that many patients who do not respond to acupuncture have an improved response when the antidepressant amytriptyline is administered in low doses.

The Treatment of Pain with Chinese Herbs and Acupuncture, a recent addition to the clinical literature on acupuncture, focuses on the manipulation of the psyche as well as of the physical body.[12] According to traditional Chinese medicine, the seat of the psyche sits in the heart and "governs the mind." Both Eastern and Western philosophies acknowledge that a healthy heart is responsible for a normal blood supply to all the bodily tissues, and that any disease or condition requires a good blood supply to improve healing.

In the past, Western medicine has typically separated treatment of the physical aspect from treatment of the psychological aspect. It is now widely accepted, however, that a patient who experiences chronic pain is best treated by a multidisciplinary team of therapists. The regimen should include acupuncture because of its ability to make a valuable contribution to both the emotional and the physical well-being of the patient. It is a welcome shift that Western medicine seems to be aligning itself with the Eastern consensus regarding the necessity for treating the whole person in every condition, especially pain.

A Testimonial

The following comes from a forty-four-year-old female patient who was diagnosed with trigeminal neuralgia that caused facial pain, toothache, headaches, and neck pain:

On 17 February 1998, my only brother died very unexpectedly. He committed suicide, something no one in our family could come to terms with easily. I have speculated a lot about the true reasons for his actions; I have blamed myself for being obtuse and disinterested; I have felt humiliated, shocked, angry, disbelieving, sad, anxious, and heartbroken. I have been through virtually every emotion in the book, including depression.

Overall, I believe my healing process has progressed well. There were, however, serious repercussions for me physically. In August 1998, I had problems with digestion. I couldn't eat properly, I had constant diarrhea, I lost weight, and I generally felt unwell. I had a gastroscopy, which revealed stomach ulcers. The situation improved with the relevant medication. At the beginning of November, I started to experience toothache, at first in only the two lower molars; then the pain spread to all my teeth, and my whole face felt very tight and tense.

I went to the dentist, who could not find the problem. The general practitioner administered anti-inflammatories. I was sent to the face and jaw specialist. He diagnosed grinding of the teeth as the cause of the problem and made a bite plate . The bite plate, however, caused severe aching in my facial muscles. It was recommended that the dentist perform three root canal treatments—which increased the pain! The dental treatment continued over the next year, with the dentist trying to change my bite, but there was no improvement.

By August 2001, my teeth were aching, pulling, and spasming. They felt like they had a life of their own! My face felt stiff, especially the left side. There were spasms from the side of my head across the left side of my face. It felt to me as if everyone could notice that my face was stiff and pulling askew. In desperation, my doctor referred me to a neurologist. The brain and sinus scans were clear. The neurologist ultimately diagnosed trigeminal neuralgia, probably caused by a virus. I had suffered from shingles six years previously, which caused pain in the center of my forehead and hairline that spread across my left eyebrow and around my left eye. The earlier virus may have resurrected itself due to the tooth-grinding and jaw-clenching. Antiepileptic drugs were prescribed to ease the muscle spasms, and I was referred for physiotherapy and acupuncture.

The acupuncture improved my overall well-being and the management of my facial pain and toothache. I was taught to meditate, exercise, and use electric currents. I am still on medication, but I feel less discomfort and have less trouble falling asleep. My face feels less stiff, and I rarely get the intense spasm across the left side of my face and neck. There are times when I am not at all aware of my face or teeth, which is a great achievement. My pain score used to be eight out of ten. Now

I often achieve two out of ten. What an amazing improvement!

As a physiotherapist, I had the privilege of spending time with my patients and communicating with them, something many health professionals in other fields are unable to do because of time constraints. My profession also allowed me to use the modality of touch, which, as we know, has great healing qualities. But it was only when I began to use acupuncture on my patients that I realized I had the capacity to treat both the wounded psyche and the ailing human body. It is with profound gratitude that I observe this ancient healing art becoming an accepted part of contemporary Western medical culture and practice.

CHAPTER 8

ELECTRICITY CAN HEAL

Life is driven by electrons. An electron going round is a little current, and thus what drives life is a little current.

—Szent-Gyorgi

I have alluded several times in this book so far to the use of electricity in healing. The human body responds to both electric currents and magnetic fields. This makes sense because electricity is the most basic form of energy in nature, and every living cell is constantly exposed to the earth's magnetic field. This chapter explains how electrical currents work in the body, and it describes several treatment options that utilize these mechanisms. The next chapter also discusses a treatment that utilizes electricity, modified direct current (MDC).

The term "electrical stimulation analgesia" refers to the relief of pain by electric current, a phenomenon made possible by the human body's responsiveness to electricity.

The nervous system itself produces an electrical transmission. Changes in polarity occur within a nerve cell, stimulating an action potential along the nerve fiber after depolarization of the cell membrane. The application of an external electric current interacts with this transmission and affects both local tissues and the whole nervous system.

Electricity has been used as a treatment for centuries. According to various researchers, electricity is the driving force for many reactions—both beneficial and disadvantageous—within the body.[1,2] The ancient Greeks used fish that emitted an electric current to ease joint pain and headaches. And over the centuries, humans discovered that magnetic fields from lodestone also relieved various ailments.

Many more studies have been done on the value of electric currents in human health, and new studies are being conducted on an ongoing basis to explore the different types and frequencies of currents that help patients with pain and healing.

Patient Comfort Preferences

"Patient comfort preference" refers to my observation that certain patients prefer a particular treatment because it "feels good" to them. There seems to be a relationship between "feels good" and "makes better." I will often ask my patients what treatment they prefer when they treat themselves; their answer may indicate to me at a scientific level the specific electrical treatment that I should administer to improve or increase their pain relief. For example:

- If a patient tends to rub, bang, beat, or vibrate an area that is painful, it may indicate that the A-beta nerve fibers, when stimulated by the above activities, produce pain relief as a result of the release of beta-endorphins (natural opiates).

- If hurting or needling an area brings relief, it may indicate that the A-delta or C nerve fibers are producing neurotransmitters, such as enkephalins, to relieve the pain.

- If heat, from a hot-water bottle or heating pad, for example, helps pain, it may be stimulating the A-delta fibers and the thermoreceptors (nerve fibers that respond to heat).

- If the patient cannot bear to touch the area due to increased pain, as in the case of sunburn or a painful scar, then touch should be avoided.

Patients often seem to have an instinctive knowledge of the stimulus that will help their condition. The patient may be correct in his or her preference; it is therefore incumbent upon the therapist to determine which electric currents mimic these effects in a sophisticated and possibly more effective manner, to produce the maximum benefit for the patient.

The compatibility of electric current with the human body is not surprising, as the body functions on electrical energy before it becomes biochemical. Cells contain ions (magnetically charged atoms or molecules) that carry either a negative or a positive charge. Therefore, very weak electrical circuits (measured in trillionths of an ampere, or amp) are continuously being made across cell membranes, and there is always a potential difference in polarity on either side of a cell membrane. A difference in polarity causes constant movement into or out of cells, and the movement, which always occurs from negative to positive, produces chemicals that maintain homeostasis (balance) in the body. In fact, the body and brain function as both an "electrical station" and a "chemical factory." When the body malfunctions—for instance, it has a swollen arthritic joint—the electrical circuits are sluggish and the chemical substances are inadequate or ill equipped to precipitate healing processes. It makes sense to "kick start" these processes by administering the specific electric current that will activate a healing response.

Advances in the use of electric currents include the development of treatments that have certain effects on the specific nerve fibers that impact particular pain conditions. Therapies utilizing these advances must be employed whenever possible to help pain sufferers.

What Happens when Electricity Is Applied?

About two-thirds of the body is water, roughly half of which is found in the cells. The cells can be likened to tiny batteries, each with a potential current of approximately four pico-amps (four trillionths of an amp).[3] As mentioned above, electrical current moves from negative to positive. When a cell's "sodium gates open," sodium ions move across the cell membrane into the cell, and potassium ions move out. This mechanism, known as the sodium pump, changes the polarity (depolarization) within and outside the cell. As a result, an action potential takes place at a certain level, a nerve impulse is initiated, and the cell repolarizes once again. It is a complex exchange of activity that relies on the release of adenosine triphosphate (ATP).[4,5]

This constantly ongoing cellular activity can be adversely affected by application of a harmful current (electrocution), by cellular damage, or by disease. However, the administration of a beneficial electric current will positively affect the body by

◆ assisting the processes of healthy cells

◆ healing damaged tissues

◆ possibly altering disease processes

Once changes in polarity have taken place and electrical currents have been initiated, a host of chemical substances degrade and others are produced. This permits all the physiological processes of the body to perform their specific activities.

A normal nerve impulse is a wave of electrochemical activity that passes along the nerve fiber using stored energy in the form of ATP. It takes place as a result of a reversal in the membrane potential from – 70 to +30 millivolts, which occurs very briefly (for one millisecond) and spreads along the nerve fiber. ATP, often called the energy currency of cells, provides energy for the building of cell components, for stimulating the sodium pump action, for the transmission of nerve impulses, for muscle contractions, and for DNA synthesis, among other activities. Essentially all endogenous chemical reactions stop when there is inadequate ATP.

When the body is functioning normally, cells' bioelectrical activity proceeds in an ordered and regulated fashion. Once injury or disease occurs, however, normal flow of electrical current in the region is disrupted, impeding intra- and intercellular transmission. The body produces an immune response to correct these cellular imbalances. As previously mentioned, applying an appropriate microcurrent can stimulate this natural healing processes.

These electrical and chemical reactions are present even in our thought processes. They take place in a highly specialized manner in every system of the body, producing, for example, neurotransmitters in the brain, anti-inflammatories at the site of the injury, substance P (a pain enhancer) in the spinal cord, hormones, and many other substances. Due to the omnipresence in the body of these processes, electric currents can be used therapeutically to

◆ reduce inflammation and swelling

◆ strengthen muscles and improve mobility

◆ improve wound healing

- decrease pain by increasing endorphins, enkephalins, melatonin, and serotonin locally, in the spine, and in the antinociceptive (antipain) areas of the brain

- improve circulation

- affect cell metabolism

This is a list of benefits that can be produced in cases of injury, trauma, pain, and, possibly, disease. It is also possible that electric currents may be used to maintain good health; modified direct current (see Chapter 9) has been utilized for this purpose.

The most powerful benefits of electrical treatments are as follows:

- They have nil, if any, side effects.

- They are nonaddictive.

- They may reduce medication requirements.

- They can prevent chronicity.

- They are economically viable.

- They improve quality of life.

Electrical Treatment Options

Most patients are unaware of the possible benefits of electrical treatments—or even of their existence. I believe such information should be available to everyone. Many of these treatments are easy to locate and use, cost less in the long term than medication, and offer the patient independence and control. Not everyone responds to every electrical treatment, but many people certainly benefit from this approach.

The rest of the chapter describes some of the main options for treatment with electrical current. After reading about these thera-pies, you, the patient, will begin to have an idea of which ones can potentially minimize your pain and improve your quality of life. You will be able to discuss the various options with your therapist, and to get advice on the best regimen and positioning of electrodes for your specific pain problem. There is no need to be fearful of applying electric currents to your body. Currents that are used therapeutically are of low voltage and frequency and can do no harm, especially when specific precautions are taken (e.g., if you wear a pacemaker).

Electroacupuncture

Electrical stimulation of acupuncture points produces chemical substances in both the area of stimulation and the central nervous system. Research studies by Becker in the 1980s found that[6]

- electrical fields exist along acupuncture pathways

- electrical stimulation promotes tissue regeneration as well as bone and wound healing

Throughout the ages, traditional Chinese acupuncturists have recommended stimulating these points by hand, either slowly or fast, in a clockwise or counterclockwise direction, which creates electric currents or magnetic fields. The direction of the stimulation will bring about either sedation or stimulation of the points. These early acupuncturists lacked our present knowledge of the physiological effects of acupuncture on the central nervous system, yet they understood the value of its effects on their patients.

It is now known that stimulating acupuncture points appears to activate sensory pathways from the local region to the spinal cord and brain. It interferes with the pain messages arising from the periphery, depending on the frequency of stimulation. (See Chapter 7 for a detailed discussion of the effects of acupuncture.) Recent studies have revealed that low-frequency stimulation of acupuncture points (i.e., at a rate of 1–4 Hz) produces natural opiates—the beta-endorphins. These effects on pain are slower, yet cumulative, and they outlast the treatment. The higher frequencies, particularly 100–200 Hz, produce rapid pain relief by stimulating the production of other neurotransmitters, such as serotonin, dynorphin, and norepinephrine. Previously, this treatment was regarded as short-lived because it was thought to produce pain relief only for the duration of treatment. However, the latest trends in electrical stimulation place stronger emphasis on higher frequencies for activating more effective and sustained pain-blocking mechanisms.

When stimulating acupuncture points, it is recommended that a low frequency be used for the first ten to twenty minutes, followed by a high frequency of 200 Hz for the next twenty minutes. The most effective length of stimulation for electrical acupuncture is between thirty and forty-five minutes. Following this method will stimulate the different types of endogenous neurotransmitters and opioids.

Many patients are unable to produce serotonin. In these cases, it may be more successful to try to access the opiate (endorphinergic) system to relieve the pain.

Application of the higher frequency (200 Hz, or at least above 100 Hz) produces a contractile and relaxed feeling that mimics the sensation and effects of transcutaneous electrical nerve stimulation (TENS; see below). The areas best treated with this frequency are muscular regions, such as the back or knee. Lower frequencies (4 Hz) will produce shorter contractions, which are useful in conditions of both pain and stiffness, such as the Ba Xie points between the fingers and in other regions for arthritis or trauma.

Transcutaneous Electrical Nerve Stimulation (TENS)

TENS is a treatment that reduces pain by affecting the pain pathways. The pain is relieved at the local site (where the pain is experienced), and pain information is prevented from spreading to central sites in the nervous system. TENS is administered with a device called a TENS unit. As the word "transcutaneous" in the name implies, the current passes through the skin.

Today we have a sophisticated understanding of a "gate" in the spinal cord that can be closed to incoming pain signals by the application of TENS currents. In the 1960s, research on the spinal gate theory demonstrated that stimulation of the large, A-beta fibers (touch fibers) activated the inhibitory circuits present in the dorsal horn (substation) and thus blocked transmission from the smaller fibers (A-delta and C fibers) on the periphery.[7] These large fibers have a lower resistance to electric current than the smaller fibers and thus transmit impulses much faster. More recent research has indicated that the most likely mechanism for pain control via TENS is the blocking of activity in the segment of the spinal cord responsible for pain, supplemented by descending inhibitory pathways.[8]

The use of TENS has evolved and become more widespread since the 1960s. The treatment is successful for some, but not for all. This is not unexpected, as there is never one treatment that will always help every person. However, it is disappointing that more people have not benefited, because the *correct* use of TENS often turns out to be the best treatment modality patients have ever tried.

TENS is relatively inexpensive—a typical device costs less than one hundred dollars—and it can be easily performed at home. The patient is able to control all aspects of treatment, such as the positioning of the electrodes, the intensity (strength), the pulse width, the mode of current, and the duration of application.

TENS is primarily a pain reliever, but sometimes a painful condition is only pain driven, and once the pain is relieved the condition itself subsides. TENS produces no side effects. Most people are able to use TENS, but it is *not* recommended for those with a pacemaker, especially a demand pacemaker. Placement of electrodes in certain configurations and over certain body parts should also be avoided, specifically: placement of opposite polarities (negative and positive) on the temples; placement on the front of the neck (carotid artery), which can cause hypotension (low blood pressure); placement over the uterus of a pregnant woman; placement over a recent fracture site (where the vibration may cause pain). Irritation of the skin may occur from allergic reaction to the elec-

trodes, from unstable electrodes, or from prolonged use of TENS; however, new electrodes rarely damage the skin. There is no danger of skin burns from the electrodes, as there is no concentration of polarity under either of the electrodes. (See Appendix B, "Treatment with TENS," for specific information on using the TENS device.)

Some patients may be referred to as "complete TENS responders." Judging from clinical experience and from a study, it seems that at least 10 percent of patients, especially those with a condition that is pain driven (possibly neurogenic), may achieve 100 percent improvement in their pain *and* their condition.[9] With the correct positioning, frequency, and duration of treatment, this figure may even reach 30 percent. It may seem that 10 to 30 percent is a small number of patients, but if only two or three treatments of TENS are necessary to attain complete pain relief, it is an excellent result indeed!

Patients who do not respond completely to the treatment are referred to as "partial TENS responders." They may achieve 60 to 80 percent relief from their pain. Because pain is decreased, quality of life is improved, and use of medication may be reduced, TENS can be considered another useful coping mechanism for these patients.

Up to 20 percent of patients experience no pain-relieving response to TENS, possibly due to

◆ a poor endorphinergic or serotonergic system

◆ previous injury by electric current (electric shock)

◆ dislike of the sensation of electric currents

◆ a lack of belief in this treatment modality

Twenty percent is a relatively small number and is similar to rates of nonresponsiveness for all other treatment modalities. It also implies that 80 percent of patients will respond to TENS with some degree of pain relief. It is therefore worthwhile for most patients to undergo a trial of TENS as a treatment for pain. However, my clinical experience has also demonstrated that it is counterproductive to continue applying TENS to patients who do not respond or who develop increased pain.

My own experience with TENS commenced in 1989 when I attended my first acupuncture course. TENS was utilized for electroacupuncture by attaching wires to the needles. Many patients responded to the low-frequency stimulation. I became totally convinced of the effectiveness of TENS when I used it under the instruction of the presiding orthopedic surgeon in a private clinic as a stand-alone modality, with the electrodes placed directly on the painful site. The clinic treated patients with acute back pain or any unusual chronic-pain condition. The only treatment I was permitted to administer was high-frequency TENS. We applied it over a period of at least three days. Initially, I was concerned that the treatment would be inadequate. To my amazement, however, many of the patients responded so well that after a few days the only other necessary treatments were back hygiene and exercises. Over the seventeen years I have been using TENS, I have developed a great respect for it.

Children respond particularly well to TENS. A study by Stilz et al. indicated success-

ful treatment with TENS of unrelenting pain as a result of reflex sympathetic dystrophy (now known as complex regional pain syndrome) in children.[10] My experience in treating children has corroborated these findings. It is postulated that children respond well to TENS because a child's nervous system has not been exposed to many years of different pain experiences. The nervous system has a memory, and previous pain experiences dictate present responses.

Many conditions, such as backache, give the impression that the conditions or limitations must improve before pain can occur. However, pain relief in and of itself often has a profound impact upon the actual condition and in some circumstances may change all the other factors. This is not always the situation. With TENS treatment, many conditions change (improve) dramatically when the pain is alleviated, yielding improvement in movement, swelling, color, and temperature, among other symptoms.

It is important to mention that most earlier research recommended that TENS be used at "high" frequencies of between 50 and 80 Hz (or 70 and 150 Hz) for a period of twenty minutes. Recently, however, many researchers have examined the value of using even higher frequencies (above 150 Hz) and for longer periods (at least forty minutes) for greater effectiveness.[11]

Research from 2003 indicates that in certain circumstances patients may lose their responsiveness to TENS due to increased tolerance of the endogenous opioids that are released with the therapy.[12] This reaction may take place after three days, is less noticeable with high-frequency TENS than low-frequency TENS, and may be reduced by

concomitant administration of other analgesics. It is also noted that the degree of increased tolerance may be reduced if TENS is
discontinued after three days and then rein-
stated after another three days. Intermittent
periods of TENS may then become more beneficial.

Patients who have been on consistent administration of morphine may fail to respond
to TENS without a modification of their drug
regimen to accommodate TENS. Tolerance to
morphine therapy is a well-known phenomenon. Therapists and patients should not despair if TENS is unsuccessful, as adjusting
or adding medications and modifying how
TENS is used may improve results.

Other substances that are widely distribu-
ted throughout the nervous system, such as
cholecystokinin octapeptide (CCK-8), may impact upon endogenous endorphin-modulated
analgesia by blocking the effects of morphine
or TENS. New studies will investigate the administration of CCK-8 antagonists in combination with TENS and/or acupuncture to improve the efficacy of these treatments.

Dorsal-column stimulator devices (TENS-
type) that are implanted near the spine to
treat intractable pain states are used at a
minimum of 600 Hz. Therefore, it may be
postulated that the higher TENS frequencies
now advocated (200 Hz) may produce even
greater improvements. Perhaps if more patients had an opportunity to use a device
with a higher frequency, the results would reveal more TENS responders. It may be necessary to urge manufacturers to produce devices with the requisite frequencies that have
been shown to be more advantageous in
pain relief.

Direct Current

This section briefly summarizes the physiological principles underlying the use of direct current in therapeutic settings. The next
chapter, on modified direct current, explains
the treatment in more detail. In fact, it is
modified direct current that is most often used
therapeutically, as unmodified, or constant,
direct current may cause tissue damage.

A direct current (DC) is a continuous current that passes in one direction only. A negative current is transmitted to the body via
wet sponges or electrodes, which causes negative ions to be repelled into the tissues and
to move toward the positive electrode, resulting in formation of acids. The positive ions
are repelled into the tissues to move toward
the negative electrode, resulting in formation
of alkalines. This process, called electrolysis,
creates changes in the underlying tissue that
affect the whole system. If misused, electrolysis may cause damage to or destruction of
tissues.

Direct current is different from TENS in
that it alters membrane stability. TENS al-
ternates polarity without creating changes
in the underlying tissues, as there is no net
charge or buildup of different substances at
the end of the impulse.

Modified direct current is one of the most
restorative electrical treatments available.
All electrical interactions in our bodies that
drive physiological processes are direct current, and the human body is highly responsive to weak electrical and magnetic signals.
Application of modified direct current can reduce inflammation and improve circulation,
thereby relieving pain. It may benefit many
conditions where inflammation is present,
including many disease processes and viral

inflammation of joints or other structures, as well as circulatory problems, such as those caused by everything from venous ulcers to injuries causing bruises.

Neuromuscular Electrical Nerve Stimulation (NMES)

Neuromuscular electrical nerve stimulation (NMES), a muscle-stimulating current, is mainly used in a therapeutic environment. However, many patients have heard of this treatment through its association with toning the muscles and slimming the body. It may be more famous in some countries for its use in beauty salons than its use in pain clinics!

Sometimes called functional electrical stimulation, NMES is important for reestablishing strength in weakened muscles. Strengthening muscles often relieves pain. Once an area of the body is injured or diseased, it atrophies from lack of use (because using it is painful). Weakness sets in very quickly, which may contribute to further pain. Strength provides support for painful areas. Back pain, for example, usually gets better with an exercise regimen tailored to the individual patient (Pilates exercises are especially useful for helping back pain). However, sometimes exercise alone is not enough to retrain muscles, such as in an ankle sprain, when the calf muscles quickly become wasted. This leads to lack of coordination and strength and often perpetuates the injury. In many such cases, NMES can help to augment an exercise program.

NMES is another treatment that has become portable, adaptable, and comfortable. It offers major benefits when integrated into a treatment program for rehabilitation. It is commonly used for the following purposes:

◆ To treat disuse atrophy (may even be used in the elderly to improve frailty and coordination)

◆ To increase and/or maintain range of motion

◆ For muscle reeducation and facilitation

Use of NMES can reduce the duration of rehabilitation, thus lowering health-care costs and returning the patient to gainful employment or independence.

According to Munsat, Mc Neal, and Walters, following NMES, human muscles have shown changes in the muscle fibers and in metabolism.[13] Results from a group of patients using NMES after knee surgery to repair the anterior cruciate ligament indicated that their quadriceps muscles had greater capacity for aerobic metabolism—that is, the muscle had improved circulation and therefore received higher levels of oxygen in the blood vessels around the knee, which improved healing. In another study of twelve patients after major knee surgery, six subjects received NMES in addition to physical therapy. These subjects demonstrated increased levels of muscle activity and less muscle wasting during the period of immobilization after surgery.[14]

NMES also has value for patients with pain. Many patients with pain in the limbs, especially those with complex pain syndromes, may respond to muscle stimulation, especially when other treatment has failed. NMES may assist these patients by giving them visible proof that their muscles are contracting (seeing is believing), or by reducing their fear of muscle contraction and movement. Especially for patients with complex pain syndromes, NMES should be offered with great care and under the supervision of a therapist as it could irritate nerve endings. Any electrical treatment that increases pain or irritates nerve endings should be discontinued.

It is postulated that NMES relieves pain via the following mechanisms:

- Muscle spindles contain A-beta fibers, the stimulation of which elicits neurotransmitters or endorphins.

- Stimulation of muscles also activates the A-alpha fibers, which have a faster conduction velocity and therefore a more immediate impact on the brain than the A-beta fibers. The improved movement increases circulation, affecting the metabolism of the muscles.

- Muscles contract after activation of the motor area in the brain through an automatic pathway of nerve activity. Muscles work together in opposing pairs: Every movement involves the action of an agonist muscle and an antagonist muscle. NMES stimulates both groups of muscles, thereby activating the motor pathways that reach the brain, improving coordination and strength in the limb.

Another term for NMES is faradic current, named after Michael Faraday, who invented the original machine. A device delivering sequential faradic current, an updated version of one originally developed by Sir Charles Strong at least twenty years ago, is used as a treatment on animals, especially horses, as well as on humans. It produces motor stimulation (via muscular contraction) that is more tolerable than most other faradic-stimulation therapies. The electrode may be moved over different areas of the body during the procedure, which is not possible with other faradic devices. This allows the user to identify the exact source of the pain and improves circulation and pain relief.

The sequential faradic current device is used to treat painful joints, muscles, and ligaments and to strengthen muscles. The areas most often treated are the spine and muscles that have been sprained or torn. The effect on the spine is to mobilize the joints and improve circulation; the effect on muscles is to reeducate and strengthen them and to improve circulation. This treatment has profound effects on pain and mobility, especially in areas of the body that are difficult to treat, such as the thoracic spine.

NMES has also produced improvement in patients with stabilized spinal cord injuries. It has assisted with dissipating hematoma and extravasation (bleeding and fluid collection) around the spinal cord, relieving pain and stimulating innervated muscles.[15] It has been observed that, in some cases, scar tissue from the original spinal injury encapsulates the capillaries, which may have some impact on healing in the spinal cord and on resultant paralysis. It is important to treat these patients as promptly as possible after the original injury. Some practitioners have also used the device on patients who were immobilized after a fracture, in order to reduce the rehabilitation period.

Other uses for NMES include the following:

◆ Spasticity management in patients with hemiplegia, paraplegia, or multiple sclerosis via contraction in the antagonist muscle of the spastic muscle (patients have shown relaxation of the spastic muscles, demonstrated by increased range of motion and improved function)

◆ Orthotic substitution (i.e., as a stimulus to paralyzed or weak muscles, eliminating the need for a brace or orthosis)

◆ Treatment of idiopathic scoliosis to strengthen the weak muscles that are opposing the tightened, shortened muscles

◆ In athletes, augmentation of motor recruitment in healthy muscle (it has been used in Russia for enhanced muscle reeducation)

Patients are encouraged to use NMES after either surgery or injury to reduce the duration of any rehabilitation program. Patients can acquire their own simple unit for muscular stimulation, the use of which will provide results including improved general circulation, increased mobility and strength, and greater independence. Patients need to be initially trained by therapists who specialize in this form of muscle reeducation, but then they may continue with their own treatment.

Microcurrent Electrical Nerve Stimulation (MENS)

Microcurrents are so small that they are not discernible to the patient. Microcurrent therapy may prove valuable to patients who are hypersensitive either to touch (e.g., complex regional pain patients) or to stronger currents such as normal direct currents or TENS. Microcurrents can normalize sensitivity and improve cell metabolism and healing at the site of the pain.

The low-amperage current used in MENS reaches between 10 and 600 microamps and is used at an intensity of less than 1 milliamp. Compare this to modified direct current (see Chapter 9), which attains a maximum intensity of 4 milliamps.

MENS has been used to promote wound healing and to treat pain and swelling. As a direct current, it may restore an electrical balance to the biological system that facilitates tissue healing and subsequent pain control.[16] Used in a therapeutic clinical situation, MENS treatment is beneficial to patients who are sensitive to touch or electrical sensation, as mentioned above, and also to children, who might be traumatized by other types of treatment.

Microcurrents were used by the Japanese after the Second World War. Practitioners would dry the skin of a papaya and then charge it with an electric current. When the papaya skin was applied to the body, it discharged a negative electrical current, producing healing effects. (Remember from the discussion of magnetic fields in Chapter 4 that a negative polarity tends to trigger various endogenous healing responses.) The Chinese also developed a material in the form of a patch that could be applied over the painful or swollen area and which produced beneficial changes in the underlying tissues of certain patients.

Sophisticated devices for delivering electrotherapy treatment have been developed in many countries. Recently, a new, more portable microcurrent device has been used extensively and with great success to treat chronic and recalcitrant pain states. Called the Alpha-Stim, it produces currents with a wide pulse and an intensity of 0.5 to 1 milliamp. It has been found to be highly compatible with the human electrical system; it comes in models that can be used to administer electrical current to either the body or the brain. The Alpha-Stim device that is applied to the body utilizes small electrodes that are barely perceptible. It has been found to relieve pain, especially the sensitivity and hyperesthesia that are present in conditions involving disturbance of the nervous system, and it also assists in improving mobility and inflammation. The model that produces current that is compatible with the brain (cranial electrical stimulation) is applied to the lower earlobes, where, in some patients, it produces a mild sensation. It has been found to relieve anxiety, depression, insomnia, and severe pain states (e.g., CRPS and hyperesthesia). If the electrodes are applied to the upper ear cartilage, improvements in spasm and mobility have been achieved in conditions such as multiple sclerosis, Parkinson's, and stroke.

In some countries (but not at this time in the United States), MENS therapy is now available in the form of a membrane that can be purchased at a pharmacy. It must be held in position with bandage or tape until it has fully discharged its current, and then it may be discarded. It is commonly used as follows:

- To treat swelling and pain, e.g., from a ligament strain

- Over an injury or contusion (bruise) site

- On any spinal area or joint

- Under a collar for neck pain

- Under a back brace for back pain

- Under a bandage for joint pain

It can also be used to treat children with injury, swelling, and/or pain.

Many patients respond positively to microcurrent therapy. It is remarkable to observe a bruise disappear or back pain diminish within hours of applying MENS.

Sympathetic Therapy

Sympathetic therapy is a patented method of administering electrical current via the peripheral nerves to stimulate the sympathetic nervous system. A device called the Dynatron STS is used to administer sympathetic therapy. It was developed for use on patients with intractable symptoms of complex regional pain syndrome. Long-term treatment (at least twenty sessions) is necessary to achieve results and to prevent and treat recurrences.

The Dynatron STS generates a multiple-beat frequency of 0 to 1,000 Hz (low to high frequencies). The current is barely discernible. A typical treatment session lasts one hour.

A retrospective study of sympathetic therapy for pain attenuation in 197 patients demonstrated complete relief in 33 percent of patients; an additional 58 percent reported mild to significant reductions in pain. Some patients reported pain relief after the first treatment, and others required several weeks of treatment.[17]

A pilot study was performed on nine patients with complex regional pain syndrome. Six patients showed improvement, with VAS pain scores reduced from 7 out of 10 to between 0 and 3 out of 10. At least one patient improved after only one treatment; others improved after six treatments.[18]

The disadvantage of this treatment is that the Dynatron STS relies on a sophisticated computer-driven program. A specific treatment is selected and programmed into the device by the doctor or therapist for each patient. According to the website of the manufacturer (Dynatronics Corporation), units are available for home use by prescription only. Rental units are not currently available. In any event, because the machine is fairly complicated to operate, a patient would require sufficient training to use it.

Transcranial Therapy

Transcranial electrotherapy passes harmless electrical current through the brain in an attempt to stimulate the release of endorphins (endogenous pain relievers). It has been used to treat such challenging conditions as constant headache, spinal cord injury, and health problems that disallow medication or invasive procedures. Some patients have better results with this modality than others, but in difficult situations it is important to explore different options.

The Pulsatilla transcranial device was developed in Israel from equipment originally designed and developed in Russia. A headpiece with moistened electrodes is applied to the patient's forehead and mastoid processes (the mastoid portion of the temporal bone, which forms the posterior part of the bone). The current is discernible, and many patients can only tolerate it at low dosages (0.5 to 1 or 2 milliamps). Treatment is administered for thirty to forty-five minutes. It increases beta-endorphin and cortisol in the brain and is used to treat headaches and degenerative diseases such as arthritis. The device has had varied results, but it is remarkable to observe changes in pain and mobility in the patients who do respond to it.

Many transcranial devices have been discontinued, replaced by more sophisticated models such as the Alpha-Stim device for cranial electrical stimulation.

◆ ◆ ◆

Different conditions and disease processes respond to different frequencies, wavelengths, and intensities of electrical current. In general, however, magnetic fields and small direct currents (especially negative currents) are beneficial to health. The scientific community continues to explore the role of electrical and magnetic fields in healing.

Laypeople in general, and pain sufferers in particular, need to become more familiar with electrical devices that relieve pain and promote healing. Clinicians and therapists need to avail themselves of knowledge of these therapies and become confident about recommending them to their patients. When considering purchasing an electrical device for self-treatment, patients should always be careful to avoid either harming themselves or incurring unnecessary expense, by first discussing their plans with their clinician or therapist. Then, armed with the requisite knowledge, they can take advantage of this healing technology and take responsibility for helping themselves.

CHAPTER 9

MODIFIED DIRECT CURRENT TO TREAT PAIN AND ENHANCE HEALTH

I n the preceding chapter, I described several different methods of using electrical currents for treating pain. The topic of modified direct current deserves to be separated from the discussion of other types of current because it has a different function from the others and introduces us to the realization that a macrocurrent that produces a specific, and at times strong, sensation can heal and change the body in much the same way as medication can. In this chapter we will learn that a modified direct current may reduce inflammation and dramatically improve circulation in cases such as contusion (bruise) and may even have effects on conditions such as ankylosing spondylitis ("bamboo spine") and osteoporosis. Other types of current do not offer these same possibilities.

Modified direct current (MDC) differs from the electrical currents described in the last chapter in the following primary ways:

♦ The shape of the wave (known as a pulse) is initially sharply and shortly rectangular; then it falls away in an exponential curve to the baseline. It then recommences, without interruption, to repeat this pulse continuously.

♦ Due to the shape of the current there is no unpleasant or burning sensation on the skin, allowing a higher intensity than is tolerated with treatment using a normal direct current.

♦ It has a longer pulse width than other currents, affecting penetration of the treatment.

♦ Sometimes a higher-intensity current has better effects in certain conditions than a current producing a very mild sensation or no sensations at all.

♦ MDC produces melatonin (a precursor for serotonin), causing patients to feel relaxed after treatment.

♦ It appears to relieve inflammation (research is unclear on this; however, patients that have inflammation improve significantly with this treatment)

♦ It produces marked and rapid changes in circulation if applied immediately after an injury that causes a contusion—the bruise may disappear within twenty-four hours.

As described in the last chapter, the term "direct current" refers to a current that passes continuously in the same direction. Direct current is widely used therapeutically to introduce medication into the body tissues (iontophoresis). All monophasic currents, however, whatever the pulse length, have the same direct current effects (TENS is biphasic and has an alternating current effect). Besides creating pain relief and muscle contractions, direct currents also cause chemical changes, owing to the unidirectional current.[1]

This process results in the removal of irritants from the area by increased circulation. The changes in cell permeability result in decreased inflammation and swelling and also have effects on autonomic system activity by reducing sympathetic tone. The facilitation of tissue-healing, therefore, takes place because of the local circulatory changes and the polar effects leading to increased cell activity.[2]

Direct current is, however, notoriously uncomfortable, as it causes a burning and prickling sensation during treatment and can normally only be tolerated for a short period of time. It is, therefore, usually applied at low intensities; for this reason it is often described as microamperage direct current.

We now understand that cells have a permeable membrane that allows ions to pass through them from the outer side to the inside, or vice versa. If a direct current is applied to the skin, an ion exchange will be facilitated in the underlying tissues and a buildup of a specific polarity will develop inside or outside cell membranes. Chemicals within and without the cell will accumulate, energy in the form of ATP will be released, and chemical substances will be formed that will affect the functioning of the cell, the tissue in the area, and the whole organism.

Action Potential Simulation (APS) Current Therapy

In the early 1990s, in South Africa, Gervan Lubbe developed a device to provide a treatment known as action potential simulation (APS) current therapy. This low-frequency electrical therapy utilizes a modified direct current that is capable of stimulating the natural cell processes at a specific, low intensity. At higher intensities it also affects the A-beta, C, and A-delta fibers (touch, pain, and temperature receptors). It is experienced as a bearable, even pleasant, prickling sensation. At higher intensities it may cause the muscles to vibrate without contracting.

APS therapy is different from most direct currents in the ways described at the beginning of the chapter. It prevents the heating or burning of tissues that can happen with uninterrupted direct current as a result of an accumulation of residual charge. The APS current is well tolerated by tissues. It may be used at low amperage to stimulate ATP production by increasing adenosine, thereby improving pain relief.[3] Decreased inflammation may also occur as a result of activation of the intra- and extracellular activities. At higher intensities it improves circulation and relieves pain and inflammation, due to the release of neurotransmitters by the facilitation of action potentials in various nerve pathways.

This particular device is probably unique at the present time due to its unusual waveform. It produces a combination of a direct and an alternating current. The pulse width is long and varies from 800 microseconds to 6.5 milliseconds, and the pulse rate varies from 0–150 Hz. The pulse is continuous and modulated and the intensity may reach 4 milliamps. For optimum release of ATP, the manufacturers recommend treatment using an intensity of between 0.70 and 1.2 milliamps. Other effects may be obtained at higher intensities. It is interesting to note that the range of frequencies produced by this device (0–150 Hz) will stimulate release of serotonin, leu-enkephalin, and beta-endorphin, among other substances, to enhance pain relief. Pain relief may also be obtained with low intensities, due to the formation of adenosine, a product of ATP release.

My clinical experience over twelve years (1994–2006) of using modified direct current (APS) on patients with various conditions yielded some surprising results that I have not observed with other electrical devices:

◆ The pain and stiffness of knee osteoarthritis were eased after just the second treatment.

◆ The pain of osteoporotic fractures in the spine was relieved after four to six treatments, when other treatments, including medication, TENS, and acupuncture, had produced no effect.

◆ Gout attacks were alleviated after one or two treatments.

◆ With just one treatment, rehabilitation was accelerated after the normal period of immobilization following a fracture. Movement increased and swelling rapidly decreased.

◆ After two treatments, patients with ankylosing spondylitis experienced alleviation of pain and improvement in mobility, effects that were sustained long after treatment ceased. (Ankylosing spondylitis, also known as "bamboo spine," is a condition in which the vertebrae fuse together, causing stiffness and often severe, permanent forward bending of the spine.)

◆ In some patients, and with certain conditions, only one treatment was required to relieve symptoms permanently.

◆ Bruises and soft swelling were often rapidly reduced with one or two treatments.

◆ A patient with damaged vocal cords, resulting from a resolved viral laryngitis that caused an inability to speak above a whisper for two years, completely recovered after four treatments.

◆ Wounds from varicose ulcers and burns improved visibly after two or three treatments.

Research on APS

APS is used in many countries, but so far formal studies have only been published in South Africa. These studies are summarized below:

1. In 1997, a double-blind, placebo-controlled, randomized study was performed on twenty patients at the Pain Control Unit, National Hospital, University of the Free State, in Bloemfontein. It was part of a larger study of seventy-eight patients with chronic back pain who all demonstrated radiological evidence of osteoporosis. The project was aimed at determining the neuro-hormonal consequences of APS therapy on beta-endorphin, leucine enkephalin (leu-enkephalin), melatonin, serotonin, and cortisol. Blood samples were collected, and standard laboratory techniques and radioimmune assays were used to determine the hormone concentrations after APS therapy.

   The results demonstrated increases in the serum concentration of melatonin after the second treatment, and in leu-enkephalin after the fourth treatment. Beta-endorphin concentrations decreased after five treatments, and serotonin and cortisol levels remained within normal limits after six treatments. These results indicate that APS treatment triggers the release of specific neurotransmitters that relieve pain. Another positive effect was the maintenance of normal cortisol levels, indicating that there may be no increase in sensitivity of nerve endings that could occur with increased levels of cortisol (the primary stress hormone involved in the fight-or-flight reaction).[4]

2. Patients with chronic backache as a result of osteoporosis were included in a randomized, patient-blinded, placebo-controlled study to evaluate the clinical efficacy of APS therapy. This study was conducted at the Pain Control Unit, Department of Anaesthesiology, University of the Free State, in Bloemfontein. Seventy-six patients participated in the study, forty-three in the APS group and thirty-three in the placebo-control group. Each patient received treatment every second day for sixteen minutes, for a total of six treatments. Visual analog scale (VAS) evaluations were performed immediately before each treatment, reflecting the pain situation in the previous twenty-four hours. The conclusion was that APS therapy could be an effective treatment for chronic backache in the osteoporotic patient.[5]

3. A randomized, single-blind study on ninety-nine patients with osteoarthritis of the knee was conducted at a physiotherapy practice under the supervision of the Pain Relief and Research Unit, Department of Anaesthesiology, Baragwanath Chris Hani Hospital, University of the Witwatersrand. The study compared the effectiveness of APS therapy on pain relief and mobility with TENS and placebo, and also determined the most effective duration and intensity of APS treatment. Although the groups were small, researchers concluded that treatment with both APS and TENS demonstrated positive effects. Research statistics revealed that APS used at high intensity for only eight minutes produced a significant improvement in night pain and knee flexibility; this improvement continued one month after the last treatment.[6]

4. Various studies have been undertaken at the Department of Physiology, School of Medicine, Faculty of Health Sciences, University of Pretoria, by Van Papendorp and others. These studies demonstrated that APS therapy increases beta-endorphin and leu-enkephalin in patients with pain, as well as ATP production in cultured cells. There were also measurable changes in signal transduction in both in-vitro and in-vivo systems.[7]

Several unpublished studies have also been conducted.[8] In 1994, a study was performed on forty patients at the Rheumatic Diseases Unit of the Department of Medicine, University of Cape Town. These patients all had osteoarthritis of the knee and needed total knee replacements. The first group of twenty patients received active APS therapy, and the second group of twenty patients received a placebo control. The study concluded statistically that two applications of APS therapy reduced self-reported pain and early-morning stiffness to a highly significant degree. There was, however, no follow-up procedure to determine whether patients enjoyed any persistent benefit from the treatment.

A general practitioner made an assessment in his practice of the effects of the APS device on the treatment of painful musculoskeletal conditions in five hundred people. In many patients he found improvement in pain relief, reduction of swelling in inflamed joints, and improvement in mobility. It was also noted that patients tended to use fewer nonsteroidal anti-inflammatories, narcotic analgesics, and steroids while undergoing APS treatment. The researcher found positive effects in many other conditions and areas outside of the musculoskeletal system. Overall, the quality of life improved for many patients.

Additional Clinical Observations

◆ Positive personality changes occur. Often, patients who arrive for treatment are irritable, angry, and depressed, due to their pain. Upon completion of treatment, they exhibit mood change, becoming more communicative and relaxed, even smiling.

◆ The treatment has successfully been utilized to improve sleep and reduce jet lag, results caused by an increase in melatonin.

◆ The treatment has been used to maintain good health through daily application of electrodes over the spinal region, or on the hands and feet. Some patients report improvements in blood pressure, reduced cholesterol, reduced joint pain, increased energy, and improved bowel and gynecological symptoms.

◆ Application of treatment over the spinal region either daily or intermittently affects the somatic and the autonomic nervous systems, resulting in a feeling of well-being.

◆ Second-degree burns appear to be relieved after two treatments. The skin is less painful, and a rapid change is visible in the epidermis as inflammation decreases.

◆ Visible changes in the device's intensity display take place spontaneously during treatment, due to the immediate interaction between the current and the treated tissue. The display may register a low intensity in a swollen and painful knee, even though the dial on the device is turned up all the way. As the treatment progresses, intensity may spontaneously register higher readings, possibly indicating changes in the swollen joint as resistance to the electric current decreases with reduction in the swelling.

◆ It was discovered that the APS device is able to measure electrical resistance in the body, which may provide an indication of the state of health in a non-injured person, or of the status of a diseased or injured area. The test, which is called the Fox Energy Test and was developed in 2001, in Melbourne, Australia, can be administered after treatment to a painful site to measure any resulting energy change. If a change has occurred in the energy reading, it may indicate whether or not application of MDC has provided a benefit. The same indicator may also be used to test the efficacy of other treatment modalities.

◆ If MDC is administered at a low intensity, it stimulates ATP production and improves cell metabolism and tissue health. If it is administered at higher intensities, it relieves pain by increasing the production of endorphins and other neurotransmitters, improves circulation, and reduces swelling.

◆ The temperature of a limb that feels cold may increase after treatment, or the temperature of one that feels warm may decrease after treatment.

◆ Many patients report that their whole limb feels lighter after treatment.

◆ Treating the spine (to produce general systemic effects) and the painful joint simultaneously may increase treatment benefits.

◆ If nerve conduction is facilitated with MDC, it may have beneficial effects on the ability to strengthen muscles.

Using MDC Therapy

For specific information about treatment with MDC, see Appendix C.

Indications for MDC treatment include any mechanical or pathological disturbances of the nerve, muscle, soft tissue, or bone, whether they result from physical injury/trauma or from pathological causes, such as inflammatory or disease processes. In addition, as mentioned, general effects (overall well-being) can be obtained when MDC therapy is applied to the spinal region or to the hands and feet. Any patient may improve after only one treatment. No further treatment may be necessary.

The negative electrodes are always placed on the pain site(s), or on the area responsible for the problem. It is more beneficial to treat the region actually affected by pain or disease (the area of pathology); however, if neurons in the region are oversensitive, it may initially be necessary to treat areas removed from the actual pain site. Treatment may be administered to the area of the spine that supplies nerves to the area of pathology. Furthermore, it has been noted that in certain patients, some local arthropathies (disorders of the joints) such as ankylosing spondylitis and osteoarthritis actually respond more favorably to a spinal treatment than to local application.

General MDC treatment to the spine has been utilized for diseases or conditions including multiple sclerosis, stress, jet lag or sleep impairment, irritable bowel syndrome, gynecological pain, and peroneal pain. Few studies have been conducted on the above treatments, but many anecdotal reports exist from both doctors and patients who have been surprised by the potential of MDC therapy. Still, it is important to acknowledge that application of any treatment must be undertaken with caution and with a goal of promoting healing, and that experimentation that may injure or harm a patient should be avoided.

Treatment can be applied for a maximum duration of thirty-two minutes. Treatment times of four, eight, or sixteen minutes are common.

MDC therapy may be used in combination with other modalities, including:

- Ice pack

- Heat pack
- TENS placed above or below the MDC region
- NMES placed above or below the MDC region
- Acupuncture needles in the area of the MDC electrode
- Electroacupuncture (via TENS) either within or in close proximity to the MDC region
- Acupuncture needles connected directly to the MDC, utilizing very low amperage

The above is only a partial list. Any other modality may be used before or after MDC treatment. With the use of MDC therapy it may prove unnecessary to apply as many modalities as are usually required in a course of physiotherapy to obtain optimum effects.

If MDC is used in conjunction with any other modality, it is possible to administer MDC treatment either before mobilization or rehabilitation, to facilitate improved mobility and compliance, or afterward, to deal with soreness that may result from a therapeutic intervention, especially mobilization.

CHAPTER 10

MULTIMODAL APPROACHES TO CHRONIC PAIN

Multimodal treatment is the use of more than one modality or medication in the treatment of a single condition. If a patient consults the doctor for a case of influenza, it is not uncommon for the doctor to prescribe a selection of different medications for symptoms of nasal congestion, fever, coughing, and infection. This is a multimodal approach to treatment.

Medication that assists pain is always a consideration and, in some cases, a necessity. If the patient experiences side effects from medication, or if none of the medications that have been tried help the condition, it may be necessary to explore other options. The most advantageous choice of treatment for any patient is a speedy resolution attainable without medication, through a nonharmful electrical, magnetic, or other approach.

Patients who suffer from pain may also experience other symptoms, such as inflammation, swelling, and stiffness. The best approach to relieving any symptoms is to eliminate all aspects of the problem. Simultaneous treatment of pain with TENS, inflammation and stiffness with acupuncture, and swelling with a modified direct current will expedite an effective result. Most uncomplicated conditions—for example, sprained back muscles—are resolved with a few physical treatments. However, the patient with chronic pain does not respond as rapidly.

This chapter outlines different regimens to treat several conditions that commonly cause chronic pain. All of the conditions that cause pain could not possibly be enumerated in a single chapter (or book). This chapter demonstrates an approach that specializes in the management of pain as a primary treatment concern. Although most of the regimens outlined herein are used to illustrate treatment for specific conditions, many of them can be applied to ordinary problems, often resulting in extraordinarily rapid relief.

Whereas most of the chapter is organized by condition (back pain, knee pain, etc.), I have also included a section on pain clinics. In addition, special attention is paid to complex regional pain syndrome (CRPS). The section on this potentially devastating condition may be one of the most helpful passages in the whole book!

All of the patients profiled in this chapter were evaluated prior to treatment with a thorough history-taking, observation, and examination for pain, a lack or impairment of mobility, and other symptoms. When appropriate, all patients received the normal physiotherapy treatments of mobilization, massage, exercise, traction, etc., in addition to pain management.

General Suggestions

This section provides an overview of the different treatment modalities that exist for the treatment of chronic pain, muscle spasm, inflammation, and postural strain.

Pain

- TENS over the painful region for three days at home, for eight hours a day, or TENS (with or without a hot pack or ice) for forty minutes over the painful region during treatment in a clinic
- Modified direct current (MDC) on the painful region, with or without a hot pack or ice
- Hot pack
- Ice
- Acupuncture (with or without electrical stimulation) on the painful area, or around the site of the pain, or above and below the painful site, with or without TENS and/or modified direct current
- IMS (intramuscular needling) acupuncture to relieve spasm
- Acutouch
- Laser
- NMES (sequential faradic current)
- Microcurrent
- Gentle massage
- Magnets
- Patches of anti-inflammatory or pain-relieving material
- Creams or gels

Muscle Spasm

- Acupuncture with deep IMS, acupuncture on the painful muscles (with or without electrostimulation), acupuncture on the traditional Chinese acupoints, acupuncture on the bony spinal region responsible for the spasm
- NMES (sequential faradic current)
- Laser
- Acutouch
- MDC
- TENS
- Massage
- Creams or gels

Inflammation

- Traction to relieve compressed and inflamed nerve endings (a home traction unit may be appropriate for certain patients, especially for the cervical spine)

◆ Acupuncture into inflamed areas or joints; periosteal pecking of the bone (pecking involves inserting the needle into the soft tissue at an area where the bone is prominent, and then using the needle to gently tap on the bone)

◆ Traditional Chinese acupoints

◆ Laser

◆ Acutouch

◆ Microcurrent

◆ Gentle massage

◆ Magnets or magnetic fields (mattresses, braces)

◆ Ice

◆ Rest, support with bandaging or taping (leukotape), collar or brace, supportive pillows

◆ Patches of anti-inflammatory or pain-relieving material

◆ Creams or gels

Postural Strain

◆ Postural correction, taping to support the spine, exercises to improve posture

◆ Exercises to improve range of movement, strengthen muscles, and improve spinal stability

◆ "Back school," in order to learn improved posture and movement skills to prevent injuries and improve activities of daily living

◆ Pilates, a form of exercise that strengthens and stretches muscles, improves posture, and stabilizes the spine

◆ Hydrotherapy in a warm pool, which permits stretching and strengthening of the muscles without pain and improves painful movements by reducing the stress on joints, due to the buoyancy of the water

◆ Classes in water aerobics, Pilates, tai chi, yoga, Alexander technique (postural-awareness exercises), stretching and toning; supervised strength-training sessions in a gym

◆ Swimming

◆ Walking

◆ Back exercises (see Chapter 11)

The patient with chronic pain resulting from injury, surgery, a virus, disease, or even for no specific reason may in addition experience postural problems, sprain, strain, injury, muscle spasm, degeneration, and inflammation. These relatively common problems may become less responsive to the normal treatments because the nervous system has been damaged as a result of the chronic pain, as explained in Chapter 6.

Back Pain

Back pain includes pain in the head, neck, thoracic region, low back, and torso. Many patients who have back pain of any sort have postural problems, either in their spinal support system as a result of natural deformities, or from remaining in static positions for long periods of time. In addition, strain or injury can sprain the local ligaments, muscles, and joints. Muscle spasm may develop due to an unaccustomed positioning of the spine, muscle guarding (holding the muscle and limb protectively to prevent further pain and injury), or splinting following an injury.

Patients who sustain injuries to their spinal joints from accidents or unaccustomed strain may develop degeneration in their spinal discs (the cushions of cartilage situated between the vertebrae). As the discs get thinner, the joints grow closer to one another, and eventually bone surfaces rub together and form extra bone (osteoarthrosis).

The natural process in most spines is a tendency to fuse; the aging process itself may lead to fusion of bones in some individuals. For some patients, fusion may cause discomfort, pain, and, due to bony inflammation or compressed nerves, even referred pain (when pain is felt in a part of the body distant from the original site of injury). Others go their whole lives without the natural process of spinal fusion causing them any discomfort. It must also be acknowledged that many patients have spinal deformities or congenital or surgical fusions and yet do not experience pain.

The case history below provides an example of a multimodal regimen to treat severe back pain resulting from an unstable spine, due, in this case, to spondylolisthesis (a deformity of the neck or lower back in which one vertebra slides over the top of another): A combination of traction, exercises, a soft brace, and acupuncture will relieve the bony problem, and TENS is advocated for pain relief.

CASE HISTORY A

A female, age forty-six, with pain after a motor-vehicle accident and from multiple failed surgeries to fuse the spine at T12 and L1.

She commented that after one of her surgeries she had not been given postoperative analgesia due to a lack of communication between her surgeon and the nursing staff. She was also advised by her surgeon that she would definitely require further surgery to her neck because of degenerative disease, and that she would have to be prepared to take large amounts of medication for the rest of her life. The patient had several discs (C5/6, C6/7) that may have ruptured over time (discogenic disease), causing pain intermittently. Discogenic disease can be evaluated as a process that may occur naturally with time. The disc spaces become narrower, resulting in less cushioning and protection between the vertebrae. The vertebral joints move closer together, and changes occur on the bones as rubbing or friction occurs. This causes new areas of bone formation, called osteophytes, which, in the case of this patient, had developed centrally and laterally on the relevant vertebrae, with no instability (i.e., the spine was stable and would not move or collapse at that level). The patient had previously undergone surgery. As mentioned, a lumbar fusion was visible at T12/L1, with a curvature to one side (scoliosis convex toward the right); a wide area of vertebral bone was removed (laminectomy) at L2; and early degenerative changes were visible at L3–L5/S1, with no instability.

Daily nonsteroidal anti-inflammatories (NSAIDs) and pain relievers were prescribed for the rest of her life. She is an example of a physically and emotionally traumatized patient, due to the accident, the subsequent surgery, the lack of postoperative analgesia, and, unfortunately, probably because of negative declarations by the surgeon on her follow-up visits. She should never have been advised that she would definitely require further surgery to her neck because of degenerative disease, and that she must be prepared to take large amounts of medication for the rest of her life.

Treatment

The following treatment was administered over eighteen months:

- Gentle mobilization to the unfused regions of her spine, from cervical to lumbar areas

- Massage; IMS needling; acupuncture for stress, pain, stimulation of the immune system, inflammation, and the region of scoliosis (see Figure 10.1)

- TENS over the spine from vertebrae C2 to S1

- MDC on muscles, from trapezius to gluteals (the patient controls the intensity of the treatment by herself, a procedure often recommended because patients will accept higher intensities—i.e., more advantageous treatment—when they are able to control the device themselves)

She was initially treated three times a week, then once a week, after which she progressed to once a month for maintenance. She attended supervised hydrotherapy, back class, and Pilates for a short period only.

Home program: daily swimming, specific spinal exercises

She uses anti-inflammatories only once or twice a week, when necessary; she participates in gardening, loves cooking (which was previously impossible) and decoupage, and *enjoys her life!*

Discussion

This patient initially had no confidence in her ability to help herself or to move naturally, and she was afraid to stop taking medicine, even when she felt no pain. When she returned to her doctor a year later with improved mobility, her improvement was neither noticed nor encouraged. (Patients need constant praise for the efforts they make to help themselves, in order to encourage them to continue in their endeavors.) She was, however, given prescription medications for the following year and advised that she would probably require further surgery at some point in the future.

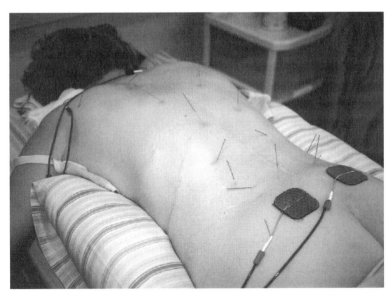

FIGURE 10.1. This patient experienced degenerative changes in her cervical spine and suffered chronic pain after failed back surgery. She is receiving acupuncture and modified direct current for her neck and back pain.

CASE HISTORY B

A female, age seventy, suffering constant pain for many months after a wedge fracture of her spine at T11 from a fall she took while her husband was severely ill.

He passed away shortly afterward. She continued to suffer pain and disability after his death. She endured constant low-back pain from her recent fall. Previous wedge fractures were also evident that had occurred spontaneously due to osteoporosis. She was therefore more susceptible to injuring herself with any future falls. She also had a severe kyphosis (abnormal backward curvature) and spinal deformity above T11. She was unable to lie on her back or drive a car.

Treatment

The following treatment was administered over one week (four treatments only):

- ◆ Electroacupuncture around the deformity in the spine, and acupuncture into the painful site (see Figure 10.2)
- ◆ MDC to the wedge-fracture area, osteoporotic regions, and pain sites
- ◆ Hydrotherapy in a warm pool to activate weak muscles and improve mobility

Discussion

This patient was soon relieved of her pain. She was mobile, able to lie on her back, and returned to driving her car. MDC therapy is renowned for the treatment of the pain of osteoporosis, even osteoporotic fractures, as it enables the patient to resume mobility. The acupuncture over the painful site and around the scoliosis improved muscle spasm and pain.

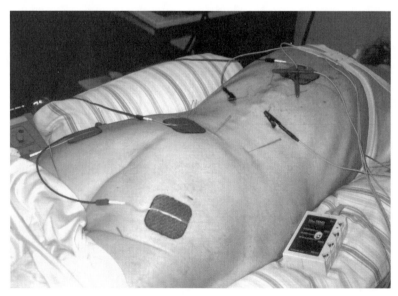

FIGURE 10.2. This patient sustained a wedge fracture in thoracic vertebra 11 (T11). She is receiving electroacupuncture on either side of the fracture site, as well as modified direct current therapy.

CASE HISTORY C

A female, age forty-six, with advanced metastatic breast cancer.

She underwent a right-side mastectomy, radiation, and chemotherapy. She experienced severe pain in the bones of her thoracic spine, thickening and scarring in her right upper chest and muscles, and a frozen shoulder (known as adhesive capsulitis and characterized by pain and stiffness in the shoulder with limitation of all the normal shoulder movements). Breathing and coughing caused pain in the front of the chest wall (in the ribs). In her back, from thoracic vertebrae T4 to T8, she experienced throbbing pain that extended deep into the armpit. She was almost unable to speak due to the sharp pain in her chest. Her right arm was swollen, and all the muscles in her arm, shoulder, and chest were tender. She was prescribed oral morphine in syrup form. She was bent forward and grimacing from severe pain, and she felt depressed and anxious.

Treatment

The following treatment was administered over three weeks, with visible improvement after the second treatment:

- Ear and scalp acupuncture for pain, stress, and anxiety
- Gentle exploratory massage to the thoracic spine, shoulder, and anterior (front) chest wall to define the regions of most tenderness (the patient enjoyed the massage; she said, "[It's] the first time I have been touched over my scars and in the painful area")
- TENS on the anterior and posterior chest wall
- Acupuncture to the shoulder to improve mobility; gentle mobilization and arm movements

Discussion

Treatment continued, with improvement in range of movement in the shoulder, general body posture, breathing capacity, and chest pain. The patient was better able to cope with her condition, and felt more relaxed and comfortable. This case illustrates that patients need to be touched, because doing so brings comfort and facilitates healing.

CASE HISTORY D

A female, age fifty-eight, with pain from failed back surgery, postlaminectomy.

The patient had constant pain in the low back and neck; she was unable to turn in bed at night. Exercise also increased her pain. She found that regular physiotherapy only relieved her pain for a few hours.

Treatment

- Gentle massage and acupuncture for muscle spasm
- TENS centrally on the spine; MDC from the trapezius to the gluteal muscles
- Acupuncture for relaxation and to relieve stress and muscle spasm
- Relaxation, breathing exercises, visualization, and meditation
- Hydrotherapy and Pilates

Discussion

Within three treatments this patient was better able to cope with her discomfort. She required a few weeks of treatment to achieve the improved mobility required to turn in bed; she was also able to resume exercising, as doing so no longer increased her pain.

CASE HISTORY E

A female, age forty-four, with cervical headaches (caused by tension in the muscles of the neck and jaw) and facial pain (diagnosed as trigeminal neuralgia).

She complained of severe pain in the right trapezius, a headache extending into the left facial and temporal region, a tight and "pulling" feeling in her teeth, extreme sensitivity in the left side of her face, poor sleep, an inability to lie on her left side (due to her facial pain and the discomfort in her teeth), and an inability to fully close her jaw. Previous treatments she'd undergone, including orthodontics, medication, and physiotherapy, had increased the discomfort.

The patient had a marked kyphosis (abnormal backward curvature) in the upper thoracic spine at C7/T1, a rotated left upper C2, marked muscle spasm in the right trapezius, and tender and indurated (thickened) areas on the face around the lips, upper and lower jaw, and left temporal region. (When pain and nerve irritation have been present for a long time, changes occur in the area supplied by the nerve, reducing circulation and resulting in thickening or other changes in the tissue.)

Treatment

- Gentle mobilization of the occiput (the back part of the skull) on the cervical vertebrae, cervical and thoracic spine, and jaw
- Electroacupuncture to relax the spasm in the cervical muscles, facial area, and sternocleidomastoid (anterior neck) muscles
- Acupuncture for stress and relaxation
- TENS for home use
- A home program of gentle exercises, relaxation, back hygiene, and Pilates

Discussion

Although treatment over many months eased the pain temporarily, did not increase pain, and improved the patient's state of mind, it did not remove all the pain. Eventually the patient consulted with a homeopathic practitioner and discovered a preparation that eased her discomfort.

Knee Pain

Knee pain can result from many conditions, including osteoarthritis, any other type of arthritis, injury, a postsurgical procedure for knee pain (such as an arthroscopy for debridement, a meniscectomy, or lateral release), patellectomy, total knee replacement, or other surgical procedures.

Most patients who have knee pain have experienced trauma from a blow or fall that has damaged bone, ligaments, tendons, muscles, and/or cartilage. This may compromise the strength in the muscles supporting the knee and may result in poor tracking movements of the patella. Misalignment may also occur from congenital abnormalities such as bowed legs.

Sports, being overweight, and age may eventually damage the patellofemoral joint and the femoral/tibial plateau in previously injured patients, producing arthritic changes and leading to muscle weakness in the quadriceps, pain, or inflammation. As the joint degrades with age, debris such as loose bone fragments or tissue collects in it, potentially impeding mobility and increasing pain, especially when the joint is "locked" in certain positions, such as in a bent position (flexion).

Many patients who have had knee surgery, whether minor or major, don't respond well. Some have more pain after the procedure than before. Hence, many orthopedic surgeons may be reluctant to investigate knee pain unless there is a flagrant problem that requires repair. The reason for the pain may be an aberrant functioning of the nervous system that supplies the knee area, which may have been traumatized by injury, surgery, or persistent pain. Genetics may also play a role. An estimated 10 percent of the population has inherited a tendency to develop chronic pain in any area of the body. The knee may become vulnerable to complex regional pain syndrome (CRPS), especially after surgical disturbance and possibly due to genetic factors. Normally CRPS strikes the peripheral joints, such as hand, wrist, foot, or ankle, but under certain circumstances it can affect the knee.

The most beneficial approach to treatment of any knee injury (or, indeed, to treatment of injury anywhere in the body) is to strengthen, mobilize, and rehabilitate the area as soon as possible. That means *exercise*.

Guidelines for the Treatment of Chronic Knee Pain

Pain and Inflammation

- Ear and knee acupuncture, acupuncture in traditional Chinese acupoints, periosteal pecking of a specifically tender region
- Ultrasound to anterior, posterior, and medial joint lines and other affected regions
- Laser to painful site
- Acutouch

- MDC
- TENS
- Microcurrent
- Magnets
- Patches containing an anti-inflammatory or pain-relieving substance (for example, adhesive patches that release a dose of the anti-inflammatory agent Voltaren can be applied to the skin over the painful region; even opioid patches can be placed nonspecifically on the body to slowly release medication in appropriate circumstances of severe, unremitting pain)
- Creams or gels

Pain Caused by Muscle Weakness

- NMES (sequential faradic current) to stimulate and develop the various muscle groups surrounding the knee, particularly the vastus medialis oblique (one of the four muscles that make up the quadriceps)
- NMES combined with ultrasound or other modalities (e.g., interferential current, a medium-frequency current that treats areas deeper than the sensory/skin regions)
- Exercises with elastic bands (e.g., Thera-Band) to help support a weak knee, provide resistance to strengthen muscles, and to increase flexibility, especially in flexion
- Hydrotherapy to provide buoyancy, support, comfort, and resistance at different stages of the rehabilitation process

◆ Free exercises with or without weights (**caution:** Moving from flexion—bent knee—to extension—straight knee— with weights must be avoided, as doing so may damage the patellofemoral joint)

◆ Biofeedback, used during rehabilitation to train the motor pathways in the brain to connect with the weakened muscle, educate it, and elicit the best voluntary response from it

◆ Controlled exercises in a gym, or biokinetics with an experienced trainer (biokinetics is a science of movement that uses individually prescribed exercises to strengthen a specific muscle or group; it prevents medical disorders related to insufficient physical activity, especially when the patient has been debilitated)

◆ Cycling, but care must be taken to avoid a deeply flexed position, which could irritate osteoarthritic conditions, especially problems in the patellofemoral joint

Knee Exercises for Basic Strengthening and Mobilization

Here is a partial list of simple and effective exercises to benefit the knee:

◆ Sitting upright in bed or on the floor, with both legs extended straight in front of you, place a pillow under the affected knee. Use your hands to try to pull the pillow sideways from its location under the knee, and at the same time, resist the release of the pillow by engaging the muscles needed to press the knee down into the pillow. This is called the "tug of war"; essentially you're preventing the pillow from moving. Hold the position for ten seconds, and work up to doing the exercise ten times.

◆ With the pillow still under the knee, place both hands underneath the knee and shake the knee up and down. This helps the muscles to relax and improves knee straightening. Repeat at least thirty times.

◆ Place a large pillow underneath both knees. Pull the foot of the affected leg upwards into dorsiflexion (foot up), tighten the knee muscles by pressing the knee toward the bed or floor, and lift the foot in line with the knee as the knee is extended (straightened). Now extend the healthy knee and pull the foot up into dorsiflexion, and compare the level of elevation of the weaker leg to the normal leg. Try to lift the weaker leg to the same level as the normal leg. Hold the contraction for six seconds and repeat ten times. Do not raise the whole leg off the bed; only the lower part of the leg should be active.

◆ Now place a small pillow or a folded towel underneath the knee, and repeat the above exercise. Compare the position of both big toes as you lift the weaker leg to the same level as the stronger leg.

◆ Repeat this exercise with no pillow under the knees. Aim to lift both big toes to the same level. When you can do so, the quadriceps should have no "lag" (lag occurs when the knee's range of joint extension is full, but the quadriceps are not strong enough to hold the lower leg in line with the upper leg).

◆ Keeping the knee as straight as possible, lift the straightened leg off the bed or floor. First pull the ankle up into dorsiflexion and tighten the quadriceps muscle by pressing the patella (kneecap) toward the bed. Lift the leg ten times without resting the leg between lifts; touch the bed with the heel only each time the leg is lowered.

◆ If the above exercise is too difficult to do without help, use a rubber band (Thera-Band) to support the leg at the ankle. Lift the whole leg upward with the rubber band. On the downward thrust, resist the movement with the elastic band, causing the quadriceps to work eccentrically (in the opposite direction). This develops strength in the leg and will eventually enable the leg to be lifted straight upward without support. Repeat this exercise ten times.

◆ Use the elastic band to support and raise the leg just off the bed. Move the leg outward, providing resistance with the elastic band as you do so, and then inward, again providing resistance with the elastic band. If possible, repeat the exercise ten times without resting the leg between repetitions. Keep the foot facing upward, and avoid rotating the leg outward. The kneecap points toward the ceiling the whole time.

◆ This time with no pillow, place the elastic band under the knee. Use the band to raise the knee into flexion as high as possible. Then resist the band as you straighten the knee. This helps to flex

the knee further when it is stiff and allows the muscles to work more efficiently as you straighten the knee. Repeat ten times.

◆ Place the elastic band on the foot, and use it to help the knee bend as much as it possibly can. Then use the resistance from the band as you straighten the knee, in a movement like kicking a ball. Repeat ten times.

◆ When you are stronger, actually kick a ball, moving your knee from a bent position to a straight one. Repeat ten times.

◆ Lying on your back and starting with a straight leg, bend the knee and try to place the foot flat on the floor or bed. If you can place your foot flat on the floor or bed, you will have achieved seventy degrees of knee flexion. If you can bend your knee enough to place your foot next to the knee joint of the other leg when it is straight, you will have achieved over ninety degrees of flexion. Repeat this exercise ten times, aiming for higher degrees of flexion each time.

◆ Lying on your stomach, tuck both feet under in dorsiflexion (feet up at the ankles, toes on the bed). Now lift the knees off the bed as you straighten the legs. Compare the weaker leg with the stronger, and aim to lift the weaker knee to the same level as the stronger knee; this helps to straighten the knee. Repeat ten times.

◆ Lying on your stomach, toes pointed, bend the stiff knee. Place the stronger leg behind the lower leg and use it to help flex the knee further. Don't force too strenuously. Next, resist with the stronger leg as you straighten the knee. Let your feet drop over the edge of the bed to enable you to straighten the knee as much as possible. Repeat ten times.

◆ Sit on the edge of the bed, feet on the floor. Use an elastic band on the foot to support and lift the stiff leg. Pull the ankle upward into dorsiflexion, then straighten the leg until the foot reaches the same level as the knee. Continue practicing this exercise until the leg is strong enough to do it without the assistance of the elastic band. Also use the elastic band to resist the opposite movement as you bend the knee. Repeat ten times.

◆ Sitting on the edge of the bed, lift the foot from the floor and swing the lower leg from side to side like a pendulum. Next, rotate the lower leg clockwise and then counterclockwise. The pendulum and rotatory movements help to improve flexion (bending) of the knee. Repeat each movement five times.

◆ Sitting on a chair, bend the knee to a comfortable position. Keeping the foot firmly on the floor and the knee stationary, slide your bottom forward on the chair, allowing the knee to bend. Repeat five times.

◆ Standing, gently step forward with the affected leg. Put your weight on the leg, and bend the knee as far as possible. Straighten the knee and then bend it again. Do this at least five times, trying to increase the bend each time.

Joint Stiffness

Stiffness may occur in any area of the body that has moving joint surfaces, for example, the spine, jaw, or limbs. The causes are varied. Sometimes a joint is unable to reach its complete range due to a disease such as osteoarthritis, which causes the cartilage to diminish, fluid to develop, and small cysts to grow on bony surfaces or soft-tissue surfaces. Changes may also occur in both the soft tissue and the bone around and within a joint, as happens, for example, in rheumatoid arthritis. Joints may be damaged by injury, lack of use (which leads to weakness and can result from chronic poor posture), or pain due to muscle spasm and inflammation.

Here is a list of treatment modalities that may assist with joint stiffness in any area of the body and from any cause:

◆ Mobilization

◆ NMES (sequential faradic current)

◆ Ultrasound in different positions, especially flexion if the joint is stiff in this position

◆ Ear, scalp, or local acupuncture

◆ Plum-blossom needling (a specialized acupuncture technique; see Appendix A)

◆ Modified direct current

◆ Acutouch

◆ Magnets

◆ Exercises (especially in warm water), hydrotherapy, water aerobics

◆ Stationary cycling

Pain Without Nerve Damage

Nerve damage in this context means nerve disturbance. If the nerves are not abnormally irritated, the response to treatment will usually be rapid and without complications.

Here is a list of treatment modalities that may assist in the treatment of pain in any area of the body if there isn't any nerve damage:

- TENS for three days, for eight hours a day, or for at least forty minutes; can be combined with heat or ice
- Ear, scalp, or knee acupuncture
- Modified direct current
- Laser
- Acutouch
- Magnets
- Creams or gels
- Patches of anti-inflammatory or pain-relieving material
- NMES (sequential faradic current) or regular faradic strengthening
- Exercises, especially in warm water

CASE HISTORY F

A fourteen-year-old male, who participates in gymnastics, suffering chronic pain in his left lateral heel.

He was unable to train for weeks due to pain suffered during weight-bearing activities and during dorsiflexion of the ankle during tumbling activities. He also developed an aching pain after these activities. He experienced no pain with normal walking. Previous physiotherapy had irritated the condition. On examination, there appeared to be an indurated (hardened) and grainy region palpable over the lateral and inferior edges of the calcaneus (heel bone). His foot was overpronating, causing a slight increase in leg length. (Overpronation, or flat feet, is a common biomechanical problem that occurs when a person's arch collapses upon weight bearing.)

Treatment

- Relaxation acupuncture was administered.
- A press needle was inserted into the ear for seven days. (A press needle is a tiny acupuncture needle that is pressed into the body or ear and is either withdrawn after a treatment or left in place for a few days, secured with a plaster. The continuous application activates the site of insertion and promotes healing.)
- He received laser and MDC to the affected area, and acupuncture to the calf muscle (K 3, Sp 6, GB 34, UB 60).
- Two magnets were placed over the grainy and indurated areas for five days.
- The patient visited the podiatrist, who made an orthotic to correct the overpronation.

After three treatments, the condition was over 90 percent improved (9.5 out of 10 on the visual analog scale), and the patient was able to train effectively. Therapy was discontinued after the fourth treatment.

CASE HISTORY G

A twenty-five-year-old female, a professional ballet dancer, experiencing chronic pain over the navicular bone (located on the front of the foot) of the right foot and in the extensor hallucis tendon (which extends the big toe).

For five months she'd endured severe pain after rehearsals and performances. She did not respond to conventional physiotherapy (normal mobilization, massage, ultrasound), rest, or anti-inflammatories.

Treatment

Two treatments of

- relaxation and ear acupuncture
- laser and MDC therapy to the painful region
- acupuncture to the leg and foot (Sp 6, K 3, St 36, Liv 3)
- application of four magnets (800 gauss each) for five days, positioned with the north pole of the magnet on the foot's painful site

The patient reported a 70 percent improvement and was able to return to rehearsals and performances. The therapy continued for about a month, until the condition cleared.

Complex Regional Pain Syndrome (CRPS)

Another heading for this section might reasonably be "Pain with Disturbance of the Nervous System." This difficult problem, which manifests with pain and circulatory symptoms, is mostly found in the peripheral joints (the ankle, foot, wrist, elbow, hand, or even the knee), but it may be present in any other area that becomes unusually painful. CRPS, formerly called reflex sympathetic dystrophy (RSD), has puzzled clinicians and pain scientists more than any other condition. It was first described in 1864 by American Civil War surgeons. Currently, medical professionals believe that CRPS is caused by some minimal type of nerve injury, yet sometimes it occurs spontaneously, with no known previous injury. It causes profound suffering, and if it is not relieved in its early phase it may lead to permanent disability.

CRPS most often presents after accidental injury, sometimes even after surgery. It may also result from a medical intervention, for example:

- An overly tight plaster of Paris or other type of splinting
- Manipulation under anesthetic
- Intravenous infusion
- A tourniquet applied during surgery
- Surgery, such as an arthroscopy, a patellectomy, the excision of a neuroma, total knee replacement, amputation, or other surgical procedures
- Investigation, procedures, and examinations by a doctor or therapist

CRPS may also result from diseases such as diabetes, neuralgia, spinal cord injury, cancer, AIDS, or even a myocardial infarction. Repetitive strain and occupational overuse may also be causal factors.

Patients can develop this condition for totally unknown reasons. In fact, it seems to occur spontaneously in 26 percent of sufferers. Previous history may, however, reveal an old injury, even in another area of the body, that healed rather slowly. If a family member had a problem with excessive pain in a joint and circulatory symptoms after an injury, it may point to a genetic factor that predisposes a patient to this type of problem.

Caution: Know the Signs!

At any time after an injury, or after a limb has been placed in any type of cast to limit movement for any reason, if the limb feels uncomfortable, or if it develops unusual or severe pain, tingling, or any unusual symptoms and/or swelling and/or immobility, especially in the fingers or toes, it may indicate the onset of CRPS. *The patient* must *consult the doctor as soon as possible to reevaluate the condition, or to remove or replace the cast. If it is not caught and treated as soon as possible, the situation may either cause CRPS or exacerbate an existing case of CRPS.*

Symptoms

Important: If any condition causes any of the following discomforts, consult a doctor as soon as possible to limit the condition, relieve the pressure or stress in the area, and treat the pain:

The *pain* may manifest as severe, unrelieved by rest, burning, throbbing, twingeing, sharp, continuous, constant, or unrelenting. It may refer proximally (upward), or the patient may use other unusual descriptions of the pain and discomfort.

The *motor* symptoms may manifest as decreased range of movement, stiffness, muscle spasm, wasting and hypotonia (lack of tone), tremor or fasciculation (trembling of muscles), atrophy leading to tissue changes, or osteoporosis.

The *sensory* symptoms may present with parasthesias (tingling and numbness), hyperesthesia or allodynia (sensitivity to touch or movement), and hyperalgesia (increased responsiveness to pain).

The *sympathetic* symptoms may demonstrate inflammation, temperature and color changes, swelling, sweating, goose pimples, skin changes, and a decrease in nail and hair growth, followed by an increase in growth.

The *psychological* consequences of such pain may be depression, anxiety, suicidal thoughts, lack of confidence, giving up hope, and unusual behavior patterns. A patient of mine who had CRPS wrapped his limb in plastic wrap to prevent the air from making contact with the skin.

There may also be an *aversion* to touch, heat, cold, wind, and air conditioning.

Often, not all of the symptoms present themselves; still, it is best to treat any symptoms as soon as they appear. The problem with CRPS is that if it is left untreated it may become irreversible. On the positive side, however, CRPS responds well to treatment; relief can be obtained if it is treated in its early stages.

Treatment Principles

The treatment will follow the same protocol as that recommended for Case History H, below. Patients with CRPS in their hands or feet usually respond well when treated with electric currents in water, notably MDC (see the diagrams in Appendix C). MDC allows the whole limb area to be treated, and the patient is able to move and exercise throughout the treatment. Stimulating muscles in the limb with faradic current (NMES) in water is also highly beneficial for strengthening muscles, improving circulation, and relieving pain in some patients.

Initial Treatment for Pain

The first treatment for pain can include the following:

- Ear acupuncture and protocol for sympathetically mediated pain (sympathetically mediated pain emanates from the disturbance of the sympathetic nervous system)
- Scalp acupuncture and deafferentation protocol for burning pain (deafferentation pain occurs after loss of normal

sensory input to the brain; an example is phantom-limb pain, where a patient still feels pain from a limb that has been amputated)

After these points have been needled, encourage active movement of the injured area. In addition, TENS is encouraged for home use, if possible.

Continuing Treatment for Pain

After the initial treatment is completed, ongoing treatment can consist of the following:

- Acupuncture above and below the painful region, and on distal points for pain
- TENS, either above the painful site, above and below it, or on it
- MDC, usually on the whole limb
- Laser on the painful site
- Acutouch near the painful site
- Microcurrent around the painful site

Treatment of Motor Symptoms

- Ear and scalp acupuncture to improve mobility (the acupuncturist should encourage movement during insertion of the needles)
- Acupuncture to the muscles and nerve supply around the affected joint
- MDC
- Gentle electrical muscle stimulation when pain subsides
- Gentle mobilization, if doing so does not increase the pain
- Exercise with gentle movements, both in and out of water, and hydrotherapy, as long as it does not increase pain (warm water is particularly beneficial)

Important: Patients with CRPS must continue to move their joints and exercise their muscles. If you don't use it, you will lose it!

Treatment of Sensory Symptoms

- Ear and scalp acupuncture
- Acupuncture around the region of aberrant sensation
- Microcurrent, especially for hypersensitivity
- Acutouch around the affected area
- Laser for sensitive areas
- MDC around the sensitive area, or on the nerve supply to this region

Treatment of Psychological Symptoms

- Acupuncture for relaxation—ear, scalp, and body
- Explanation and discussion of the causes, effects, and resolution of the condition
- Visualization and breathing exercises
- Hydrotherapy
- Positive and enjoyable activities
- TENS/MDC to release neurotransmitters (to improve sleep, mood, and relaxation)

Pilot Study of Patients with CRPS

I conducted a pilot study of ten patients who were diagnosed with CRPS and had the following conditions:[1]

- Three patients with total knee replacements

- One patient with a bruised patella
- One patient with an injury to the patella
- One patient with torn muscles and ligaments in the thigh and knee
- One patient with a traumatic chondromalacia patella (softening of cartilage under the kneecap that commonly occurs following a knee injury)
- One patient with a patellectomy (surgical removal of the patella)
- One patient with an ankle sprain
- One patient with a spontaneous manifestation of pain in an ankle

Where their condition made it appropriate to do so, all the patients were tested before and after treatment for straight-leg raise, flexibility of the knee, and VAS pain score. Each patient received acupuncture, TENS, and physiotherapy. All of them experienced a highly significant improvement in all three tests. Before treatment, the VAS scores had a mean value of 7.78 with a standard deviation of 2.05. After treatment, VAS scores improved to a mean value of 0.38 with a standard deviation of 0.89, producing a statistically significant difference of $p < 0.05$.

The protocol outlined above has been used on countless patients with CRPS or any other form of severe pain. Most patients experience a positive response that is repeatable upon further use of the protocol.

CASE HISTORY H

A twenty-eight-year-old, male, professional soccer player, who sustained an injury to his knee on the soccer field.

He received three arthroscopies (a procedure that enables a surgeon to view the inside of a joint) over a period of two weeks. He had undergone an arthroscopy to his other knee seven years previously. His main complaint was severe stiffness. Any attempts to rehabilitate him with normal physiotherapy and rehabilitation increased his stiffness and pain.

On first consultation, his range of movement was 60 degrees of flexion and 20 degrees off full extension. The knee was severely swollen, hard, and indurated, with many areas of tenderness in all the surrounding muscles. He limped severely and was deeply depressed, as he had been a candidate for the world soccer tour. He was taking the medication Neurontin (an anticonvulsant that is also used for the treatment of nerve pain) as well as analgesics.

Treatment

- Ear, scalp, and local acupuncture
- TENS trial for three days, eight hours per day
- MDC, massage, and gentle exercises, progressing to NMES, mobilization, and hydrotherapy

Discussion

The goals of treatment were to prevent irritation and exacerbation of his symptoms so he could progress to normal rehabilitation. Within ten treatments, he was able to flex to 110 degrees and lacked only 5 degrees off full extension. He was more cheerful and could walk normally. He was able to return to his soccer training.

CASE HISTORY I

An eleven-year-old female with pain in her left lateral ankle joint.

The referring diagnosis was CRPS type 1. (CRPS type 1 involves an aberration in nerve conduction;

CRPS type 2 indicates actual injury to the nerves in the area.)

History and Symptoms

The patient presented with generalized pain in her left lateral ankle joint that she'd experienced for three weeks. During the holidays a few months earlier, she had spent a great deal of time barefoot. When pain subsequently developed in her ankle, she was referred for physiotherapy that included ultrasound, massage, interferential current (medium-frequency current that stimulates the deeper nerves, not necessarily the skin nerves), and exercises for the ankle. Pain increased and was not alleviated by nonsteroidal anti-inflammatories. The patient was then referred for pain management.

She was sensitive to touch (hyperesthetic), was on crutches, and could not bear any weight on her foot. She had severe limitation of dorsiflexion and eversion (outward rotation). She described the pain as burning and sharp; it disturbed her sleep. The foot was cold, and the VAS pain score varied from 5 to 10 out of 10.

Earlier History

Two years previously, the patient had sustained an overuse injury in the ankle, as diagnosed by the doctor, and had been placed in a plaster of Paris cast for four weeks. The pain settled down until one year later, when general aches and pains developed in both ankles and orthotics were prescribed.

Treatment

The first treatment consisted of laser acupuncture to the ear. (Laser treatment uses an infrared laser to exert a photochemical action at the cellular level. The laser light can be used on acupuncture points because it stimulates abnormal tissue to activate its normal intercellular radiation and thus restart the healing process.) Laser was also used to treat the ankle region, and MDC was applied to the whole

lower leg to improve circulation. The patient used TENS at home for three consecutive days, eight hours per day.

After the second treatment, the patient reported a varied VAS pain score of 2–10/10. She still had pain at night, the foot remained cold, and there was a reduced and now specific region of pain in the region of the ankle's lateral collateral ligament. The mother reported a change in the child's personality, stating, "I have my child back!" The child was less depressed and more cheerful. Treatment was repeated, with application of direct current to the painful region. TENS was continued at home as before.

After the third treatment, the patient reported 0/10 on the VAS pain scale, there was full movement of dorsiflexion and eversion, normal temperature was restored in the foot, and the patient was fully weight bearing and had discarded the crutches. There was still some tenderness in the lateral collateral ligament region. The previous treatment was repeated, and direct current and ultrasound were applied to the painful region in the ankle. Rehabilitation exercises were instituted in the pool and on land to improve balance and coordination. The patient was advised to continue with the use of orthotics. Otherwise, no further treatment was required.

Discussion

This patient's condition was referred to as a "CRPS ankle." A literature review revealed a study by Stilz et al. that indicated successful treatment with TENS of CRPS in children, as mentioned in Chapter 8.[2] I have also found that using TENS to treat CRPS in children has a very high success rate. I chose to treat this patient with TENS at home for at least three days, for eight hours per day, because I have had excellent results over many years of using this exact protocol. Using this regimen, it is possible to detect "the complete and the partial TENS responders."[3] As demonstrated in the pilot study referred to above and in many clinical situations, pain relief may be obtained by using TENS for as little as two to three days, despite the length of time the pain has been present.

This patient's previous history of injury to the ankle region and then long periods without support to the foot (orthotics) predisposed her to developing CRPS. The pain became generalized, disguising the pain in the focal region. The conventional physiotherapy treatment increased pain, eventually rendering the patient unable to bear weight on the affected foot. The distressing symptoms that ensued—burning pain, night pain, inability to bear weight, cold foot, and hypersensitivity—created a change in the child's personality. She became withdrawn, miserable, and depressed. At the first session, laser acupuncture was administered to the relevant points in order to avoid creating fear or any further discomfort and to engender confidence in the treatment. Nonpainful laser treatment was applied to the local region, and a direct current was applied to the whole leg to improve general circulation in the ankle.

It is important not to increase pain during treatment of CRPS because any increase in pain or discomfort will irritate nerve endings, causing the condition to deteriorate. It was important to explain to the patient the procedures involved in the various suggested treatments and the reasons for selecting them, as well as the expected probability of success, relative to other children with this same syndrome. Doing so hopefully produced the placebo response, which relies to a certain extent on the belief system and the confidence of the patient in the treatment procedure.

After the first treatment, the patient experienced more than 50 percent improvement in the pain, as well as a positive change in personality.

Furthermore, the pain had become localized to the lateral collateral ankle ligament, which allowed us to subsequently focus our treatments there. At the third consultation, the child was pain free and had spontaneously discarded her crutches. The only additional treatment required was training to increase balance, coordination, and strength, in order to prevent recurrence.

CASE HISTORY J

A forty-four-year-old female diagnosed with CRPS following nerve injury that occurred three weeks earlier when a garden hose accidentally struck the outside of her lower leg at the level of the peroneal nerve.

The patient said, "I was angry at the time of the incident." Her anger was unrelated to the injury but rather was directed at personal matters.

The patient was unable to bear weight after the incident. The pain extended from the region of the peroneal nerve into the anterior (front) ankle joint. There was also slight pain extending into the medial aspect of the thigh. The pain was described as burning, pulling, shooting, and hot. She suffered increased pain at night. Her VAS pain score was 7/10. Other remarks made by the patient were, "I cannot sleep, and my leg is not getting better."

Observation and Examination

There was no active dorsiflexion, and all other ankle movements were minimal. The patient experienced discomfort when pressure was applied to the painful areas. There was no visible sign of injury in the region of the pain, and the patient was non–weight bearing on crutches.

Treatment

◆ Ear and scalp acupuncture, electroacupunture to the leg

◆ MDC therapy from the peroneal region into the ankle

◆ TENS at home for eight hours a day for three consecutive days

After the second day of TENS, during the second and last treatment, a VAS pain score of 0/10 was recorded, dorsiflexion and all other ranges of movement in the ankle were normal, the patient had discarded her crutches, there was no night pain, she was sleeping through the night, and no further treatment was necessary.

Discussion

If treatment had been initiated that increased her pain, such as ultrasound, mobilization, or even massage, her condition may have been exacerbated. After two treatments of TENS, a pain-blocking modality, distal acupuncture, and nonirritating direct electric current to the local region of pain, the symptoms improved. During the first treatment after the ear acupuncture, the patient was able to move the foot into dorsiflexion and eversion without difficulty. She was also able to ambulate more comfortably.

On arrival for the second treatment, there was no further pain and full movement had been established. It was decided to cease further treatments. She described her mental state at the time of the injury and was able to understand that stress could have irritated and exacerbated the injury. She decided to consult further with a psychologist to deal with various life issues.

CASE HISTORY K

A female, age thirty-one, who'd had a hemangioma (a benign tumor filled with small, tightly packed blood vessels) removed from her right knee in 1976, a bone cyst removed in 1993, a bone graft and biopsy in the interim period, a total knee replacement (TKR) in 1998, and a second TKR in 2002.

She presented with severe burning and aching pain, and stiffness and wasting of the muscles surrounding the right knee joint. Her extension was limited: fifteen degrees of full extension and seventy-five degrees of flexion. She also complained of pain in the left leg in the same areas as that in the right knee (mirror pain).

Treatment

Over the previous two years the patient had been treated with many different therapies, including acupuncture (using a protocol for deafferentation and sympathetically mediated pain), electroacupuncture over the painful site in the knee and leg, modulated direct current, ultrasound, massage, laser over the painful sites in the knee, acutouch, and muscle-stimulating currents. These treatments eased the pain but did not improve movements until transcranial electric current was added. After only three transcranial treatments, administered once a week, she attained a remarkable change in extension (negative five degrees) and easily reached ninety degrees in flexion. The quadriceps muscles began to activate (get stronger) and develop bulk.

In April 2003, the patient smilingly reported that she had just returned from a week-long holiday during which she'd gone horseback riding (her favorite sport, which she had not done since 1999). She was able to maintain a well-flexed knee, and the vibration of the horse's trotting did not create any added discomfort. Treatments continued once a week until the pain subsided and mobility returned enough to allow normal activities of daily living.

Circulatory Problems

Many patients develop injuries or diseases that affect the limbs (e.g., diabetes), potentially compromising circulation and causing varicose ulcers, pain, and sensory changes. Such outcomes can lead to lack of use or even loss of the limb.

Treatment Guidelines

◆ Always keep the limb moving, especially the affected joints, unless there is an unhealed fracture or malevolent disease process present.

◆ MDC current has profound effects on circulation, heals wounds and varicose ulcers, and relieves inflammatory pain in nerve endings.

◆ Laser heals skin wounds.

◆ Acupuncture improves circulation.

◆ Acutouch may also prove effective.

CASE HISTORY L

A twenty-eight-year-old male diagnosed with frostbite after having been stranded during a heavy snowstorm in Utah while travelling by car with his girlfriend.

They had no warm clothes or suitable shoes and only a bag of sweets for sustenance. They sat in their car for four days, waiting for help, and eventually left the car and spent five days trying to walk through the wilderness to civilization.

The young man eventually had to leave his girlfriend, who was too weak to continue. He walked an additional twenty miles before he was rescued. He recalled that the clothes covering his lower legs were frozen solid. A search party later found his girlfriend, who had died.

The patient was hospitalized for a week. He returned to his home in South Africa in a wheelchair, suffering from unbearable pain and sensitivity in the soles of his feet and toes. He was unable to move his toes or ankles or to bear weight on his feet. Understandably, he was also depressed and tearful.

Treatment

◆ Ear and scalp acupuncture (both deafferentation and sympathetically mediated pain protocols)

◆ Acupuncture for stress and sadness (Du 20, EP 1, Ren 17, Lu 7)

◆ Laser to the painful regions

◆ Nerve creams (St. John's wort, lavender, basil essential oil) for use at home

◆ MDC therapy in water to both feet simultaneously

TREATMENT MODALITIES THAT ENCOURAGE WOUND-HEALING AND RELIEVE PAIN

◆ MDC

◆ Electroacupuncture at each end of the wound, or into the tender areas of the wound

◆ Microcurrent

◆ Laser

◆ Acutouch

◆ Creams or oils (especially lavender oil, unless the wound is open)

◆ TENS for home use, or 40-minute treatments in a clinical setting

---

◆ One magnet retained for home use on painful and traumatized right big-toe joint

Discussion

The patient experienced marked improvement after each treatment. By the third treatment, he discarded his wheelchair. All movements in the ankles and toes were restored, and sensitivity was almost nil in the soles of the feet. The patient was able to discuss his ordeal spontaneously; he reported feeling much better, because his emotions had stabilized.

Wounds

Wounds can produce severe pain and discomfort. They can cause the following complications:

◆ Hypersensitivity

◆ Pain, with twingeing, shooting, sharp, and electrical sensations

◆ Infection

◆ Redness, inflammation, and thickening, which may indicate that the tissue underneath the wound has not properly healed

◆ Referred pain, which causes pain, discomfort, or tingling in the whole joint or tissue, far removed from the wound itself

◆ Delayed healing, with unhealed gaps left in the wound

Pain Clinics

Pain clinics are a fairly recent innovation. A multidisciplinary team of medical professionals who specialize in pain management work together to analyze the patient and the condition and offer different and combined treatments to break into the pain cycle. The multidisciplinary approach is necessary because the problem affects so many aspects of the patient's life, including its overall quality.

A pain clinic usually combines the skills of the following professionals:

◆ *Anesthetist:* prescribes medications and administers interventions to block the nerve sensations that cause pain

◆ *Physiotherapist:* relieves pain and stress with massage, electric currents, and acupuncture; mobilizes, massages, stretches, and strengthens taut muscle and nerve structures; educates the patient on pain management; advises on home treatments that may relieve pain (e.g., TENS, others); improves exercise capacity

◆ *Acupuncturist:* uses acupuncture needles to relax tight structures, decrease inflammation, relieve pain, improve mobility, and relax the patient

◆ *Occupational therapist:* provides activities and assistance to improve strength and mobility, especially in the work environment; may employ hydrotherapy, back classes, and postural correction

◆ *Behavioral therapist or psychologist:* helps the patient to change belief systems, thought patterns, and attention given to the pain; addresses any personal problems relating to the condition and lifestyle of the patient; program may include relaxation, visualization, and breathing exercises

Unfortunately, not all chronic-pain patients have access to, or the financial means to attend, a pain clinic, especially in the privatized health-care system of the United States. Moreover, in third-world countries, pain clinics have to rely on state funding, and the treatment of chronic pain is rarely high on the agenda.

CASE HISTORY M

A twenty-nine-year-old taxi driver from Liverpool, U.K., who was involved in a motor vehicle accident that totaled his automobile.

Immediately following the accident he experienced severe pain in the right thoracic (upper) spine (T6 to T11), severe low-back pain, and referred pain down the side of his left leg. He limped severely, favoring the left leg, and bent forward as he walked, virtually using only the muscles in the front of his legs to propel himself forward.

His severe pain left him unable to continue his profession. He could barely cope with the normal activities of daily living, and he could only sleep on his stomach, as lying on his side (on either side of his ribcage) was unbearable. He took ibuprofen and received two physiotherapy sessions involving electric current and traction, which caused numbness in both legs. Out of desperation, he began to search the Web to find some help for his problem. He read about my center for pain management and rehabilitation, and he arranged to come to South Africa for two weeks to try a program for his problem.

On first examination, he was very stiff. He had no rotation in his thoracic spine, limited low-back movements in all directions, and severe muscle spasm in the right upper back and in the whole of the low-back area. He was unable to raise his legs beyond twenty degrees, with the left leg feeling worse when he raised it than the right leg. There

was no muscle activity in his back or buttocks muscles, and his left sacroiliac joint was out of alignment. (The sacroiliac joint connects the two large pelvic—ilium—bones with each side of the sacrum, located at the base of the spine. The strong ligaments surrounding the joint can be strained and moved slightly out of position, causing backache and pain upon movement, especially walking.) He was depressed, anxious, and nonsmiling.

Treatment

The program, administered by a group consisting of three physiotherapists, a Pilates instructor, and a psychologist, included the following:

- Nine physiotherapy sessions of mobilization, massage, electroacupuncture, MDC, NMES (sequential faradism), and TENS, which was administered continuously for three days and which resulted in a partial pain relief

- Four sessions of sacroiliac manipulation, muscle strengthening, and reeducation in walking

- Six sessions of hydrotherapy to stretch tight structures, improve mobility, and strengthen abdominal muscles

- Four sessions of Pilates (enough to train the patient in a regimen that he continued at home) to strengthen abdominal and back muscles and correct posture

- Three sessions of psychotherapy

The exercise, psychotherapy, and physiotherapy at times took place on the same days.

Discussion

The patient experienced changes in mobility after four days of treatment but reported little improvement in his pain. We demonstrated the changes in movement to him, as it seemed that he had to understand and see the changes for himself in order to continue improving. At his next session, he reported that he was sleeping better at night and that his pain was easing. The psychotherapy sessions commenced at this stage.

His treatment was completed after nine days, with complete relief of all pain and restoration of full range in all spinal and thoracic movement. His ability to raise his left leg, which was limited to seventy degrees due to tightness in the posterior leg muscles (hamstrings), will eventually improve with consistent stretching of these muscles. He walked normally and without a limp. He demonstrated a changed personality and a smiling and confident countenance.

He was given a list of exercises to do and was told to contact us at any time by e-mail if he had any problems in the future. He was advised to continue with his Pilates and walking regimens and to make contact with a physiotherapist in his area, if necessary.

This patient really wanted to get well. He complied with all of the suggested activities, did his exercises diligently, and accepted the psychotherapy with a positive outlook. Still, when he arrived, he was unsure of what to expect and had almost given up hope of a complete recovery.

A program such as this one is simple and cost effective and could be managed in any country. It included simultaneous exercise and psychotherapy and increased the patient's sensory and motor input. It converted an inactive and painful patient to a mobile, more comfortable and contented person.

Each patient has a unique combination of symptoms, signs, and emotions that requires individualized evaluation and treatment to relieve pain and restore quality of life. As this chapter illustrates, each patient, together with his or her health-care practitioners, must determine his or her own path to pain relief.

On this path, the patient may begin to understand the truth of the idiom "Physician, heal thyself." We are all physicians of our own bodies. We must learn to take responsibility for that fact by helping ourselves whenever we can, and also by helping our healers help us by providing them with intelligent and useful clues. As mentioned previously, every word the doctor or therapist utters to the patient is important. Likewise, every word the patient utters to the doctor or therapist is important in helping the "medical detective" to understand the problem and offer the best solution.

CHAPTER 11

EXERCISES AND ADVICE FOR THE CARE OF YOUR BACK AND NECK

D o you know that 90 percent of all back pain can be eliminated without surgery or drugs? Do you know that most back pain is caused by constriction of muscles compressing a nerve?

Recent research at Johns Hopkins University Hospital implicates soft tissue as the culprit in 90 percent of all back-pain problems. Muscles, tendons, ligaments, fascia, nerves, cartilage, and blood vessels are all soft tissue that may be involved in back pain.[1] The muscles, ligaments, tendons, and fascia hold the bony skeleton upright. The nervous system, consisting of the brain, spinal cord, autonomic nervous system, and peripheral nerves, provides the nerve supply to the torso, arms, and legs.

In terms of back hygiene, most people's biggest problems are poor posture and lack of exercise. If you maintain good posture and regularly exercise your body, both of which this chapter aims to help you do, you will experience less strain, sprain, and injury, and you will have better circulation, mobility, strength, and flexibility, as well as a more positive mental outlook.

Physiology of Back Problems

Many people admit that they have poor posture, but they don't know how to correct it. They do not stand comfortably or sit straight. Poor posture can lead to or exacerbate myriad back problems.

Kyphosis and Scoliosis

Two congenital spinal deformities are kyphosis, which is an excessive backward curve in the thoracic spine, and scoliosis, which is a curvature of the spine to one side in the upper (thoracic) spine, lower (lumbar) spine, or both. Besides having congenital causes, either condition can also develop after an injury or accident or be the result of years of poor posture.

Kyphosis is also associated with osteoporosis, a thinning of the bones due to reduced calcium deposition, especially in the elderly, and with ankylosing spondylitis, a disease that stiffens the spine due to the destruction of the joint cartilage.

Scheurmann's Disease

Another disease that affects the spine and creates deformities or poor posture is Scheurmann's disease, which always sounds worse than it is. The end plates of the vertebra in the thoracic or upper lumbar spine fail to grow normally, mostly during puberty, producing an increased kyphosis in this region. The condition can be minimized by exercise and is not usually painful.

Herniated Disc

A disc herniation, often referred to as a "slipped disc," is a common diagnosis of a condition that typically results from injury. It usually occurs after making a bending and/or twisting movement while picking up or carrying a weight of some kind (e.g., a baby or piece of furniture).

Each disc, situated between two vertebrae, behaves like a cushion. All vertebrae have discs between them. The disc looks like an onion, with a soft inner nucleus surrounded by tough rings. If the nucleus bulges backward, it presses against the spinal cord. If the nucleus bulges sideways, it compresses the joints that arch together to form the foramen, or the hole through which the spinal nerves pass. If there is a tear in the outer rings of the disc, the inner nucleus and outer material may move out of position and compress the spinal cord, facet joint, and/or nerve tissue.

Pressure from a herniated disc creates muscle spasm and pain, and shifts the posture. The patient, unable to stand upright, may bend slightly forward. But he or she cannot bend very far forward, move the legs comfortably, or easily put on socks and shoes.

Muscle spasm occurring from other causes may create similar movement difficulties. In addition, stiffness in the hamstring muscles, which attach to the buttock muscles and permit the spine to bend forward easily, can be a culprit in loss of spinal mobility. Stiffness in the hamstrings is caused by lack of stretching before and after sports activities. It also occurs in people who have sedentary occupations and do not participate in exercise and stretching.

A disc herniation requires relief of muscle spasm as well as specific exercises to push the disc material back into its natural position. Sometimes traction can help. Once the disc moves back and the joint has stabilized, it may take six weeks for the joints to actually heal, even though the movements have normalized and the pain has diminished.

Once the disc has been damaged, the "onion rings" surrounding the soft nucleus become thinner, providing less support between the vertebrae. As the disc continues to thin down, especially as a result of hard physical labor, heavy-pressure exercises such as weight lifting, and aging, the vertebrae may grow closer together, resulting in compression of nerves and muscle spasm. Thus, strengthening and stabilizing the spine is important to protect the spine and prevent future "slipped discs" and joint pain.

Osteoarthritis

When osteoarthritis affects any area of the spine, it is known as spondylosis. The condition causes degeneration of the joints and thinning and breakdown of the cartilaginous intervertebral discs. The discs may lose their soft inner pulp and the onion rings become thinner, thereby affording reduced cushioning between the vertebrae. Bony surfaces grow closer together, causing rubbing of vertebra on vertebra. Inflammation and possible growth of spurs, called osteophytes, may occur at the edges of the vertebrae. Pressure from disc material may build up backward, toward the spinal cord, or laterally (sideways), into the foramina on either side of the vertebra. The foramina house the spinal nerves as they leave the spinal cord. From here, the nerves travel throughout the body to supply the muscles of the head, neck, torso, back, and limbs. When nerves are squeezed due to narrowing of the foramina, it may cause neurological symptoms in the limbs, such as pain, tingling, pins and needles, numbness, and, sometimes, weakness.

The spine may become compressed in the area of the spondylosis, due to collapse of disc space. Cervical joints may then fuse into positions that create a forward head posture and produce a "hump," or increased curvature at the junction of the cervical and thoracic spine. This situation can cause aching, muscle spasm, and nerve compression, creating pain and possibly tingling or numbness

down the arms. If the problem exists in the low-back region, it may produce these symptoms in the legs. Exercise, stretching, and traction will usually relieve these symptoms.

Misaligned Vertebrae

In the conditions spondylolisthesis and retrolisthesis, one or two vertebral joints are out of alignment, causing one vertebra to move slightly forward or backward against another. This situation may create tension on a nerve, resulting in neurological symptoms. It may also create instability in the spine, so that bending forward and extension movements produce pain and muscle spasm.

Again, the correct exercises that stabilize and strengthen the spine will be effective. Traction and a soft brace may also be necessary. A soft mattress and a flexible chair that does not encourage excessive arching of the back are also recommended, as extension exercises may irritate this particular condition. It may be helpful to use a chair that encourages lumbar flexion, such as a deck chair and a mattress that curves in the center to accommodate the spondylolisthesis.

Sciatica

A patient who has nerve root compression may suffer sciatica, in which pain is usually felt in the buttock, extending down the leg and often into the foot. Pain may or may not also be present in the back. The pain may move down the leg on the side, the back, or the front, depending on which nerve roots are involved. The pain may change, and pins and needles and numbness may also occur. Sciatica is not dangerous, *unless* severe, sudden weakness develops in the foot and leg, and/or bladder and bowel symptoms arise.

After pressure has eventually been relieved on the spinal nerve, any weakness will spontaneously recover over a protracted period of time, usually six months to two years. Patients need to understand that even if the nerve is released, it still remains bruised; this may continue to produce pain, tingling, and weakness as healing occurs. As healing progresses, pain and discomfort may move out of the leg or arm and into the back or neck, depending on where the nerve damage occurred. This is actually a good sign, because if pain moves out of a limb and into the back or neck it indicates that there is reduced pressure on the nerve. Usually treating the back or neck with careful mobilization will easily resolve the discomfort in the local back region. If the nerve is severely compressed, with symptoms extending into the limbs, then mobilization of the spine will only increase pain and damage and is to be avoided.

Many people grow despondent because nerve pain is very unpleasant, especially at night. Patients often become desperate and decide that surgery *must* be the answer. Unfortunately, surgery may not always produce relief, because the nerve still has to recover and heal, despite surgical intervention.

What helps? Rest, when necessary; sometimes traction and/or a soft brace; medication; electric pain relief; specific exercises; gently stretching the hamstrings; swimming; keeping as active as possible; and *patience!*

How can stretching the hamstrings help? The sciatic nerve follows the same path as the hamstrings in the posterior thigh; stretching those muscles also helps to stretch the nerve. A tight nerve root may reduce mobility in the spine and leg, and gentle stretching of the nerve will improve healing and mobility.

Correct Posture

Now that we understand what can happen to the spine with injury or disease, we will analyze correct posture and how to go about achieving it.

Most people cannot attain a perfect posture, due to different body shapes and minor differences in the configuration of the spine. Still, striving to correct the positioning of the body will improve matters. This chapter does not discuss every type of poor posture, but it does offer general guidelines to help improve posture. It also outlines easy—and easy-to-remember—exercises that can improve your back's strength, mobility, and flexibility.

Correct posture means good body alignment. This involves balance between opposing sets of muscles. Muscle imbalance occurs when muscles are persistently exercised to develop strength, without exercising the opposing muscles (e.g., regularly exercising the quadriceps without exercising the hamstrings).[2] Another cause of muscle imbalance is when one group of muscles habitually remains in a shortened position while the opposing muscles remain lengthened, such as might happen from sitting and looking at a computer all day. The opposing muscles actually become weaker.

Important! Over time, poor posture causes loss of the natural curvature of the whole spine, changing both the shape of the spine and its height. With these changes, it becomes impossible to maintain certain activities, and lifestyle becomes restricted.

Posture Principles

The head is balanced on the seven cervical (neck) vertebrae, which have a natural forward curve (lordosis). The twelve thoracic (upper back) vertebrae are positioned under the cervical spine and curve in the opposite direction. The lumbar spine (lower back) sits under the lowest thoracic vertebra; its five vertebrae also curve forward, resulting in the hollow that you can feel in the lower back. The lowest lumbar vertebra rests on the sacrum, which is solid and has a backward curve, similar to that of the thoracic spine (see Figure 3.2 on page 34).

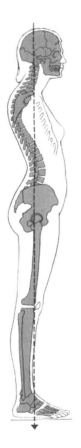

FIGURE 11.1. Imaginary line indicating good posture

The sacrum has joints on each side that allow it to interface with the pelvis at the sacroiliac joints. Although these joints move only minimally, they are affected by the muscles that maintain spinal support. Exercises that strengthen and support the pelvis and spine will affect these joints, contributing to pain relief and improved spinal movements.

Good alignment can be achieved by imagining a line extending downward from the top of the head, passing through the front of the cervical vertebrae and lower thoracic vertebrae, extending through the middle of the lumbar vertebrae and pelvis, slightly behind the center of the hip joint, slightly in front of the center of the knee joint, and slightly in front of the lateral malleolus (outer bone) of the ankle joint (see Figure 11.1).

How to Correct Your Posture

♦ Stand in such a way that you are able to see the profile of your body in a mirror. With your legs slightly apart and head upright, visualize a soda straw running in a line through the center of your body, passing from the crown of your head to your feet as described above.

♦ Rock gently backward and forward to find the center of your body.

♦ Keep your bare feet balanced firmly on the ground, feeling the floor and using all the toe and foot muscles to hold the feet in balance on the floor.

♦ Slightly relax the knees by bending them very slightly.

- Let the arms relax; drop the shoulders, letting gravity pull them down.

- With the back of the head in line with the upper back, widen the space between the ears and the shoulders by stretching the muscles of the neck.

- Lift the chin and keep it tucked in instead of poking it forward.

- Lift the rib cage, and position the center of the chest over the center of the pelvis. This helps to straighten the shoulders from the forward (slumped) position and repositions the head on the shoulders.

- Pull the stomach/abdominal muscles in firmly, to center the pelvis directly over the center of your feet.

- Grow taller. Stretch the body (the soda straw) upward until the vertebrae feel as if you are stretching them gently apart.

- Feel the tension gently increase in the muscles in your back, close to the spine.

- Maintain the hollow (lordosis) in your lower spine (keep the back straight).

- Tighten the buttock muscles gently, but do not tilt the pelvis.

- Place the tongue behind the back of the upper front teeth.

- Breathe in through the nose, allowing the rib cage to expand sideways and downward.

- Breathe out through the nose. As you release the rib cage, continue breathing and maintain the tension in your abdominal muscles.

- Start by holding the position for one minute; gradually increase to five minutes.

Take this beautiful posture with you whenever you move!

This positioning will correct forward head posture, keep the shoulders upright without straining the actual shoulder-girdle muscles, and maintain stability in the abdominal muscles. As you become more accustomed to holding this position, practice it when standing in line, or at any other opportunity that may present itself. Holding good posture is one of the best exercises you can do. It should become a daily habit.

Another aspect of posture that is worth mentioning is the effect of emotions on the body that can create changes in posture. For example, a teenage girl with large breasts may feel embarrassed and may walk with her head dropped forward and her chest hollowed to minimize the size of her breasts. If she continues with this habit, she will retain the posture for the rest of her life, causing much discomfort and even disability. If, however, she improves her self-confidence, is encouraged to hold her posture to show off her beautiful breasts, and, if necessary, loses a little weight, she will grow into an upright, active, confident, and happy person.

Another, more common problem is the typical "computer posture" adopted by people of all ages who spend many hours in front of the computer. Computer users tend to sit with the head forward, bending the lower neck (cervical spine) forward and extending the upper part of the neck backward. This is called the forward head posture. It can affect the upper spinal nerves as they become squeezed against the back of the head, producing a stiff neck, tension in the muscles, and possibly even headaches. As a result of this poor posture the whole back curves forward, giving the appearance of a rounded back. This adds to low-back pain, increases stiffness in movements, creates stress on discs and joints, and may increase the possibility of developing degenerative changes in the spine and weak muscles in the abdomen and back. The problems most commonly encountered in poor posture start at the top of the body with poor sitting position. See Chapter 3 for tips on sitting at a desk, and see below for additional tips on sitting and driving.

Exercises for the Neck

Exercises Done While Lying Down to Correct Forward Head Posture

Do each of the following exercises five times:

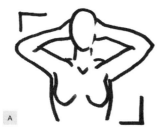

- Lying in the supine position (on the back) on the floor on a mat (see A), bend the knees and place the feet flat on the floor. Place both hands behind the neck, with elbows bent, and push the elbows flat onto the floor. This helps to contract the muscles between the shoulder blades and stretch the pectoralis muscles in the upper front part of the chest. Keep the stomach muscles firm.

- Place both hands behind the neck. With the neck relaxed and supported by both hands, lift the head forward to rest the chin on the chest, if possible. Next, lower the neck, vertebra by vertebra, onto the floor, allowing the lowest cervical vertebrae, situated at the junction of the neck with the shoulders, to touch the floor first.

- With arms by your sides, tuck the chin and press the back of the neck toward the floor, making a double chin. (Tucking the chin is called retraction.) Hold the retraction for six seconds, and then slowly relax. If the neck is too far forward to accommodate this position, place a pillow under the head to do the exercise.

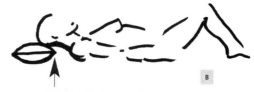

½ inch off pillow or floor

- Start in the same position as above, with or without a pillow under the head. Retract the neck, lift the head one centimeter (one-half inch) off the pillow or floor (see B), hold for six seconds, return the head to the pillow or floor, and then release the retraction.

- Holding the retracted position, rotate the neck to the left (i.e., look to the left), maintaining the retraction for six seconds. Now return the neck to the middle, maintaining the retraction, and then relax the neck. Repeat five times, and then do the same exercise to the right.

Sitting Exercises for the Neck

Do each of the following exercises five times.

- Sitting in a supportive chair and maintaining a gentle chin tuck, lift the rib cage to straighten the shoulders. Shrug the shoulders up to the ears, hold for six seconds, then slowly release the shoulders.

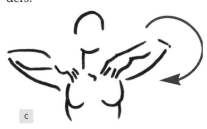

- With fingertips on shoulders (see C), circle the elbows five times in one direction, and then repeat five times in the opposite direction.

- Retract the neck, tucking the chin in. Hold for six seconds, and then relax.

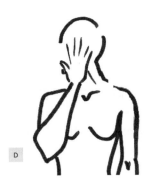

- Rotate the neck to the right (see D). Placing the right hand on the left cheek, gently coax the neck to the right as far as comfortable. Hold for six seconds, then gently release. Return the neck to the midline. Repeat to the left.

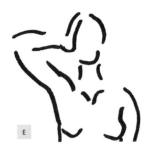

- Head facing straight in front, place the right hand against the right cheek (see E) and push the cheek against the hand without moving the head. Resist the movement (isometrically), keeping the head straight. Hold for six seconds, and then relax. Repeat with left hand against left cheek.

- Head facing straight in front, place a hand on the forehead. Without moving, use the hand to resist the forward movement of the head. Hold for six seconds, then relax.

- Head facing straight in front, place a hand at the back of the head. Without moving, use the hand to resist the backward movement of the head. Hold for six seconds, then relax.

Standing Exercises for the Neck

Do each of the following exercises three times:

- Stand with your back against a wall, tuck the chin in, hold for six seconds, and then release.

- Standing with arms by your sides, turn the head to the right, place the right hand on the left cheek (see F) and gently turn the neck as far as possible. Then stretch the left hand towards the floor,

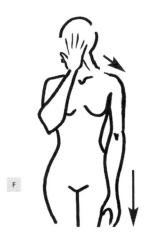

keeping the body upright. This stretches the nerves (roots) as they exit the foramina on the side of the neck. Hold for six seconds, then release. Repeat on the opposite side.

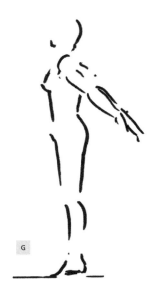

◆ Standing with correct posture, stretch the arms out sideways and backward (see G), palms facing outward, with the wrists extended backward as far as is comfortable. This stretches the nerve roots as they exit the foramina in the

neck and travel along the nerve pathways in the arms.

Tips for Headache Sufferers

Most headaches are related to a combination of neck and jaw problems and stress. Neck muscles support the head and extend into the back of the head. The head can move in all directions when joints and muscles in this region are healthy. However, if the neck is held in a certain position for some time, then the muscles become strained and tired, and the neck cannot be maintained in its normal position. Compression of joints and soft tissues, including nerves, ligaments, and muscles, occurs. The jaw muscles may also become strained due to clenching of the teeth, which can happen consciously or unconsciously, even during sleep. If a person is under stress, the muscles in all regions of the body automatically become tense, which impacts tired and weak muscles in the neck and jaw, increasing pressure on areas that may have been subject to degeneration or injury (e.g., from whiplash). Headaches result both from tension in these muscles and from compression of nerves and joints. Headache pain can be referred into the forehead and facial muscles.

Headaches and arm pain, especially pain below the elbow, may respond to gentle traction. Traction in the cervical spine (neck) stretches the neck in a manner that separates the joints (vertebrae) and stretches the ligaments to release any pressure that may be compressing soft-tissue structures, including nerves, and causing pain. The best position for traction is with the neck in flexion (bending forward), obtainable by using at least two or three pillows to support the head. This is a gentle procedure that separates the tissues only a little bit. When traction is administered for nerve root compression, ideally it is given for longer periods (at least twenty minutes) using a very light weight (three to five kilograms, or six to ten pounds). Traction can be administered in a clinic, or, if the condition is chronic, a simple and economical home traction unit can be used on the advice of the therapist.

Here are some more pointers for finding relief from headaches:

- Under the advice of a therapist, use a collar for six weeks while driving, working, and reading.

- Lie on the floor and place a thin (no more than 1.5 inches) book under the back of the head (not the neck) for five minutes daily. The book supports the back of the head, allowing the neck vertebrae to stretch away and releasing the pressure on the nerves at the back of the head.

- Correct the forward head posture and consciously maintain a good head position.

Exercises to Stretch the Thoracic Spine

The thoracic spine, which lies between the neck and low back, moves less freely than the other parts of the spine. It is necessary to stretch this region to maintain strength, balance, flexibility, and a good alignment—all of which assist with good posture.

The following exercises will benefit the elderly as well as patients with stiff thoracic spines. Do each of them three to five times.

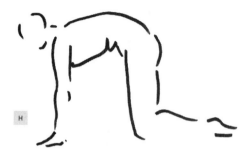

- Get into position on your hands and knees (see H). Position the body with knees directly under hips and hands directly under shoulders. Tighten the stomach muscles and maintain a normal low-back arch. Next, round the spine as high as possible, like a cat stretching and rounding its back. Hold for ten seconds, then release and return to the starting position.

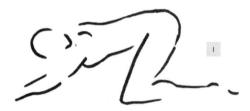

- Still on your hands and knees, stretch the hands and arms forward until the head touches the floor (see I). With the back stretched out as straight as possible, hold the position for ten seconds, and then release.

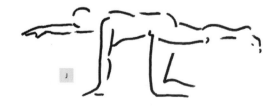

◆ Still on your hands and knees, lift the opposite arm and leg in line with the body (see J), and lengthen them away from the body simultaneously, growing longer. Maintain your balance, keep the back in a neutral position, and tighten the abdominals. Hold the head in a neutral position, not flexed or extended. Hold for ten seconds, return to the starting position, and repeat with the opposite arm and leg. This specific exercise is particularly helpful for elderly people; it improves balance in standing and walking.

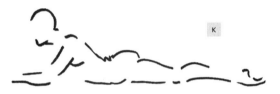

◆ Lying on the stomach (prone), lift and support the upper body on folded arms (see K). Stay in this position, arching the thoracic spine while resting on the elbows, for ten seconds. Then release.

The Low Back

The low back (lumbar spine) supports the whole spine. Most problems in this area stem from weak abdominal muscles, which create a strain on the low back by increasing its natural lordosis. This produces a highly arched lower spine and stresses the joints situated toward the back of the spinal column.

In certain people (e.g., those with osteoporosis or ankylosing spondylitis), the thoracic spine may sink onto the pelvis, creating an increased kyphosis (backward curve) of the lumbar spine and lower thoracic spine and resulting in the forward head posture.

The patient appears bent over. The result is a terrible posture that causes the abdomen to protrude and weaken because the muscles cannot be tightened or activated. The ability to arch (extend) the back is lost, and the patient cannot stand or walk in an upright position. Height is diminished, breathing capacity is reduced, and compression of joints and nerves occurs, often causing great discomfort and pain.

The two most common postures that reduce spinal mobility are an increased lordosis in the lumbar spine with a protruded abdomen, and a reduced or flat lumbar spine that has lost extension. Stiffness in the lumbar spine, during both flexion (bending forward) and extension (bending backward), hampers the movements of daily living.

The abdominal muscles work in conjunction with deep muscles surrounding the back of the spinal column; if these muscle groups work together, posture will be balanced. The back muscles hold the spine upright, and the strong abdominal muscles hold the stomach in position, allowing the lungs to expand fully. As you can see, if we don't stand correctly, we are unable to get sufficient oxygen into the lungs, which can affect all bodily functions.

The muscles that hold the abdomen in its correct position provide a complex lattice of support, which, when the muscles are contracted or tightened, is similar to having an external brace around the whole lumbar spine and stomach. The fibers of the abdominal muscles attach from the lower ribs to the pubic bone (front of the pelvis) and iliac crest (front aspect of the pelvis bones above the hip joints), each group having its own specific attachments. Contracting these muscles, especially the internal obliques, affects

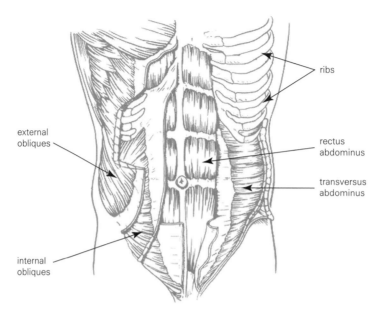

FIGURE 11.2. Abdominal muscles

the muscles and the joints in the back area. The muscles of the back cover a large area and are attached from the deep surfaces of all the vertebrae, extending in many layers until they are palpable under the skin.

When injuries occur, especially in the lumbar discs, normal lordosis is lost, possibly resulting in a permanently curved lumbar spine. This rounded curve extends into the lower thoracic spine, causing the cervical spine to hyperextend in order for the patient to see in front of himself or herself. This posture will also force the patient to walk bent forward, unable to straighten upward, which may also shorten their stature. These abnormal postures also usually shorten and tighten the hamstring muscles. Patients may lose forward flexion in the lumbar spine and become unable to touch their toes.

The following exercises will strengthen the abdominal muscles and back muscles, allow deep breathing, improve mobility in all the lumbar joints, and stretch the hamstring and quadriceps muscles and all the neural structures. They will help also prevent rotation of the pelvis, especially when the sacroiliac joints are not level.

Abdominal-Strengthening Exercises

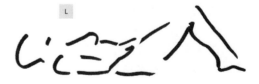

Lie on a mat on the floor (see L). Bend the knees and place the feet flat on the floor. Do each of the following exercises ten times:

♦ Breathe in, expanding the lower ribs as far sideways as possible; breathe out and flatten the ribs as you contract (pull in) the abdominal muscles. Continue normal breathing as you hold the tension in the abdomen for ten seconds. As you do so, press the back toward the floor (but do not tilt the pelvis). Press your fingers on the lower abdomen to ensure that you hold the abdomen contracted.

♦ Do the same exercise as above, but during the abdominal contraction, lift one flexed knee slowly upward, bringing it directly above the hip (i.e., bending the hip to ninety degrees). Maintain the contraction as you slowly lower the knee and place the foot on the floor. Now release the contraction. Tighten the abdomen again and then lift the opposite leg; then lower the leg and foot to the floor and release the contraction.

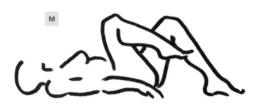

♦ Do the same exercise as above, but while contracting the abdominal muscles lift one flexed knee (see M), return the foot to the floor, *continue to hold the contraction,* and then repeat with the opposite leg. Lower the flexed knee and place the foot on the floor, and *only* then (i.e., after lifting and lowering both feet consecutively) release the abdominal contraction. **Important:** Do

not release the abdominal contraction until the second foot rests on the floor.

♦ Learn to breathe while holding the abdominal contraction. Do this by breathing, expanding the chest and the lungs at the base, then releasing the breath as you hold the contraction.

Back-Strengthening Exercises

Do each of the following exercises five to ten times:

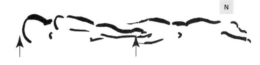

½ inch off floor   *½ inch off floor*

♦ This exercise strengthens all the muscles in the back. Lie on your stomach on a mat; rest your forehead on the mat and your arms alongside your body (see N). Lift your head and arms one centimeter (one-half inch) off the floor; hold the position, with chin tucked in retraction, for ten seconds.

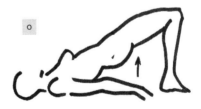

♦ This exercise strengthens the buttocks and all the neck and back muscles. Lie on your back on the mat with knees bent and feet flat on the floor. Contract the abdominal muscles and tense the buttock muscles without tilting the pelvis; then lift the pelvis and buttocks so that the pelvis is in line with the knees, if possible (see O on the previous page). Slowly return the back to the floor, vertebra by vertebra, starting with the thoracic vertebrae first, and lowering the spine until the last lumbar vertebra touches the floor. Maintain a constant abdominal contraction.

Stretching Exercises

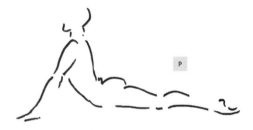

♦ Lie on your stomach on the mat, and, with elbows bent, place your hands next to your shoulders. Push your upper body upward as high as possible, keeping the sacrum area (just below the lumbar spine) on the floor and straightening the elbows to the extent possible (see P). Breathe in as you push the body up, hold the breath, extend your head back, and breathe out, allowing the low back to sag even lower and thus increasing its extension. Breathe in as you return the upper body to the floor. Perform the exercise gently at first. Then, as you increase your range of movement, extension (arching of the spine) will eventually improve. Repeat five to ten times.

Caution: If this exercise increases pain or causes the pain to move further away from the spine or into the leg, **stop immediately**!

Important: This exercise may help to push the nucleus of the disc back toward the middle/interior of the disc. For this reason it is recommended twice daily, five to ten times each session, but *only* if it decreases pain and improves movement. These specific exercises were designed by New Zealand physiotherapist R.A. McKenzie for improving disc injuries.[3]

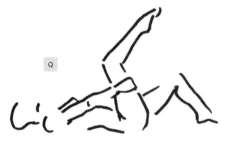

♦ Lie on your back, with knees bent and feet flat on the floor. Stretch one leg upward as high as possible (see Q); this stretches the hamstrings and the sciatic nerve. Try to straighten the knee when the leg is in the air. Return the foot to the floor, in the bent-knee position, and repeat with the other leg. Repeat the exercise five to ten times.

♦ Do the same exercise, but straighten one knee from the bent-knee position, and lower this leg straight to the floor without resting in this position; then return the leg to the bent-knee position. Repeat with the other leg. Repeat the exercise five to ten times.

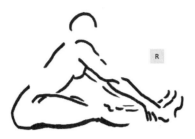

◆ Sit with legs as straight out as possible. Rest the hands on the legs, and then slowly move the hands forward toward the ankles until you feel the hamstrings stretch (see R). Keep the back straight by hinging at the hip rather than rounding through the back. Hold this position for thirty seconds. **Caution:** Avoid this exercise if you have a disc that was recently damaged.

◆ Lie on the back with the right knee bent. Place the left ankle on the right knee, support the right knee in both hands, and pull it toward the chest. This will stretch the left buttock. Hold for thirty seconds. Repeat with the left knee bent and the right ankle resting on the left knee. Support the left knee in both hands, and pull it toward the chest. Hold for thirty seconds. This will stretch the right buttock.

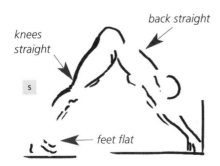

knees straight

back straight

feet flat

◆ Get on your hands and knees, with your fingers placed against a baseboard to prevent slipping. Lift your knees slightly off the floor, straighten the upper back and arms, keep the head between the arms, then lift the buttocks up toward the ceiling as you straighten the knees and stretch the hamstrings (see S). Keeping the knees as straight as possible, try to place the heels on the floor. Stay in this position for thirty seconds. Do this exercise, a modification of the dog-stretch exercise taught in yoga, once a day to stretch hamstrings and improve forward bend of the spine. This exercise improves flexion after only one try!

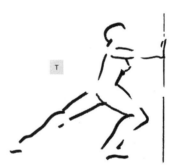

◆ Face the wall, standing about an arm's length away from it. Resting your hands at shoulder height against the wall, step forward with one leg, bending this knee and stretching the opposite calf by keeping the back knee straight and the heel flat on the floor (see T). Hold for thirty seconds and then repeat with the other leg.

◆ Standing, hold on to a rail or chair for support. Bend the left knee and grasp the left foot with the left hand (see U on the next page). Pull the bent leg behind

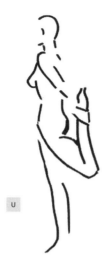

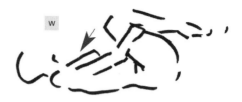

until the feet touch the mat. Place your hands on your knees and/or thighs to assist, if necessary. It is safest to do this exercise in the late morning or early afternoon (see "Tips for Movement," below).

your body, keeping the back straight. Hold for thirty seconds. This stretches the front of the thigh (quadriceps). Return to neutral, standing with both legs on the floor, and repeat with the right leg.

Flexibility Exercises

Lie on the floor on a mat, bend the knees, and place the feet flat on the floor. Do each exercise five to ten times.

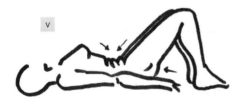

- Tighten the abdomen and contract the buttock muscles together, flattening the back into the floor (see V). This is the pelvic tilt. Hold for six seconds, and then release.

- Gently bring the bent knees onto the chest (see W), then lower the knees

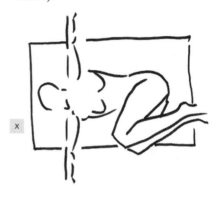

- Extend your arms out along the floor at shoulder level. Keeping the shoulders and feet on the floor, gently lower both knees to one side (see X). Return to the middle, stop, and then lower the knees to the opposite side. Return to the middle.

- Bending the right knee and keeping the left knee straight, lower the right knee over to the left as far as possible, keeping the shoulders flat on the floor. Return to the starting position, change legs to bend the left knee and straighten the right leg, and lower the left knee to the right as far as possible. Return to the starting position.

Tips for Sitting and Driving

Sitting for long periods of time decreases the lordosis in the low back, allowing it to round and sag into flexion. It places forward pressure on the discs, producing backache and stiffness. In addition, sitting in a low chair or on a couch may irritate an existing disc problem, or even create a disc problem.

Chapter 3 provides tips for sitting at a desk. You should also observe the following general pointers for sitting:

- After sitting for an hour, get up from the chair and place your hands in a supportive position behind your low back. Arch your torso backward, and then return to neutral. Repeat five times, keeping your hands in position to support your back.

- Always sit with your knees at the same level as your hips. Sitting with your hips lower than your knees causes rounding in the low back, reducing its natural lordosis.

- After driving for one or two hours, get out of the car, walk around for a minute or two, and do the back-arching exercise described above.

- Whether you're sitting in a chair or a car, use lumbar support. Roll up a towel and place it behind your back at waist level (in the small of your back). Lean back against the towel. The added support will hold the back in gentle extension instead of allowing it to sag into flexion.

- Whenever you sit down, try to keep your spine in a normal lordosis (i.e., keep the back straight). You can do this by imagining that someone has a string attached to the crown of your head and is gently pulling upward. When supported by the muscles in a lengthened posture, the spine will find its natural curvature. This is an exercise that, if practiced consistently, will become a way of life and will promote strong back and abdominal muscles. It is your *best sitting exercise.*

Tips for Movement

During the day, the compression of gravity on the body, in combination with our upright posture, causes the discs between the vertebrae to become thinner. The spine is more stable in the afternoon, making it less vulnerable to injury than it is first thing in the morning. During the night, the discs do not have the pressure of the body weight upon them; in addition, they naturally absorb water, becoming slightly puffy by morning, which increases the risk of injury. Flexion (bending forward) first thing in the morning may damage a swollen or puffy disc by placing pressure on the spinal cord and nerves. Take care of your vulnerable spine when bending forward right after you wake up. Follow the guidelines spelled out below, in "Bending Forward."

Many injuries occur during the simple movements of getting in and out of bed, standing up from sitting, bending over, picking articles up from the floor, and lifting heavy items. Here are some pointers for practicing good sleeping-posture habits and good back hygiene when performing the following activities of daily living:

Lying

◆ Sleep on a firm mattress with good support.

◆ Sleep should rest the spine. If pain increases while sleeping, it may be due to an uncomfortable mattress.

◆ Many people have back pain at night due to joint inflammation, possibly caused by inflammatory joint disease, a condition unrelated to the comfort and quality of the mattress. Electrical currents and/or anti-inflammatory medications may help ease this pain.

◆ Unfortunately, the bed that supplies good support for one individual doesn't always do the same for another individual. People should have a mattress that supports their spine, even if it doesn't necessarily support their partner's.

◆ If a person wakes up with pain, it is possible that, during the sleeping hours, the spine was compromised and became injured.

◆ People who are of lighter weight will require a softer mattress than heavier individuals. A lightweight person who has a comfortable and supportive mattress and still feels pain on waking should try placing a foam mattress (eggshell) on top of the original mattress.

Side-Lying

◆ Most people are more comfortable lying on their sides. While doing so, a supportive roll may be used to fill the space between pelvis and rib cage. Women have larger hips than men; adding support to this space may increase back comfort while side-lying. A rolled towel may be secured around the waist; it will not move during changes in sleeping position.

◆ Lying with knees bent and a pillow between the knees provides comfortable back support. (People who prefer to lie on their back may find that a pillow or two under the knees provides comfort.)

◆ When rising to sitting from lying, roll on to the side, bend the knees, drop the feet over the edge of the bed, sit upright by pushing yourself up with the arm that lies underneath the body, and steady yourself with the opposite arm.

Sitting to Standing

◆ Use a good lumbar support when sitting for long periods, as previously discussed.

◆ Move forward on the chair or bed until the feet are situated on the floor slightly behind the knees. If necessary, use the hands on the seat or arms of the chair or bed to push the body upward; use the thighs to propel the body upright, maintaining a normal lordosis (i.e., keeping the back straight).

Standing to Sitting

◆ Reverse the above process. Stand with the back of the legs against the seat of the chair, and, if necessary, place the hands on the arms of the chair. Retain the lordosis (keep the back straight) as you use the thighs to lower the buttocks gently onto the chair.

Standing Up with a Weight

◆ In most cases, this would apply to a parent lifting a child as she or he stands up from a sitting position. Seat the child on the lap facing your chest, and stand up as described above (sitting to standing). Encourage the child to place his or her arms around the lower part of your neck or to hold on to your body, usually at the shoulders.

Bending Forward

◆ Maintain the lordosis (keep the back straight). Bend the knees and then bend the body forward at the hips to reach the floor. This protects the low back by sharing the load of bending with the knees and hips.

◆ On returning to the upright position, retain the lordosis and use the thighs to lift the body upright.

Lifting

◆ Bend as advised above, grasp the article in your arms, and hold it close to your body. Retain the lordosis, and use the thighs to lift the body upright.

◆ To lift a load from the floor, retain the lordosis, maintain a firm footing and a wide stance, and have a secure grip on the load. Bend the knees, and place yourself as close to the load as possible. Straighten the knees and lift steadily. Do not jerk, shift your feet to turn, or twist your back.

◆ To lift a table, for example, or another heavy object, stand close to the object, bend the knees, and lift it off the ground. Then move it with assistance, if possible, to another position. Retain the lordosis and the bent knees until the load is once again on the floor.

Walking

Walking is one of the most important exercises for the spine. In the modern world, more people spend most of their time sitting in cars, watching television, or working at a desk than walking. If we do not spend some of our time walking, we will lose a vital movement that retains the natural ability of the human spine to move in an upright posture. The human spine is designed to hold the body upright and to permit the body to extend as we walk. If the spine is stiff and cannot extend properly, how would it be possible for the individual to stand up straight or walk comfortably?

Besides the suggested exercises for improving back extension, the simple and cost-effective exercise of walking does the same thing and at the same time improves posture and therefore quality of life.

Progressing to More Advanced Types of Exercise

Many helpful exercises and methods of exercising exist. I am sure that many new and innovative exercises will be designed and discovered in the future that will greatly benefit back pain and stiffness.

If there is injury or chronic pain, the patient must be carefully guided along the path to wellness with suggestions that are comfortable and that resonate with him or her. Posture correction is necessary to assist the spine in retaining its normal range of movement in all daily activities, either while overcoming the effects of injury or during normal living. Good posture also facilitates a better quality of life.

Exercising in a group offers great social and psychological benefits. Perhaps look for an exercise group that begins with an informative back class to reinforce knowledge and to make sure that the exercises or movements are performed correctly to prevent injury. It is recommended that relaxation, visualization, and meditation techniques be included in these classes to heal all aspects of the personality.

After the back class, the client may progress to water aerobics or Pilates, whichever he or she prefers. Either will encourage the patient to learn to move in a friendly, comfortable, safe, and nonmedical environment, and perhaps to join a group of people who have had similar problems and are now exercising for enjoyment and good health.

The teacher of water aerobics or Pilates has to correct and monitor the clients and understand each person's weaknesses, strengths, and capabilities before encouraging him or her to join a group session. The patient is now moving away from the role of "patient" to that of "client"—someone who has the strength and capacity to choose a suitable exercise regimen for him-/herself.

Hydrotherapy

In this context, hydrotherapy, which is the use of warm salt water for the treatment of stiff and painful joints, is recommended. Hydrotherapy is also used in the treatment of disease, where patients are immersed in baths of water infused with herbs or other substances chosen for specific purposes.

Hydrotherapy provides a supportive, comfortable, enjoyable environment in which the patient finds all the movements easier and less painful to perform. This is due to the buoyancy of the water. When the patient can move easily and achieve a range of movement that was impossible on land, the weaker and stiffer regions of the body strengthen, enabling the patient to move more easily on land. The patient may also learn to relax (and let go of tense muscles) in the water.

Hydrotherapy strengthens, stretches, relieves pain, improves relaxation and sleep, and provides confidence in balance and movement. It is successful in helping to treat arthritic ailments and sports injuries, and it also helps with stress reduction.

Pilates

Pilates is a system of exercise that improves flexibility through the toning and strengthening of the muscles. It involves a series of controlled movements that strengthen the "powerhouse" of the skeletal support system: the abdomen, lower back, and buttocks. Part of the program involves teaching the mind to engage with the body in performing movements correctly; through this experience, the mind develops a new awareness of muscle function and control.

The benefits of Pilates include a long, lean, toned physique, weight reduction, improved posture and flexibility, reduced stress and tension, prevention of injury, rehabilitation, and pain relief. It can lead the patient carefully along the road to recovery and produce confidence in the exercise process of life.

Tai Chi and Yoga

Other recommended exercise classes are tai chi and yoga. Tai chi has long been respected for its healing and therapeutic value. Sometimes called a moving meditation, it consists of a sequence of movements practiced very slowly and with concentration. It exercises all the major muscle groups, lubricates the joints, and stretches ligaments and neural structures. It also improves balance by incorporating specific weight-shifting postures that incorporate turning, twisting, spiraling, and squatting movements, accompanied by deep breathing. It improves circulation and oxygenation and energizes and calms the mind.

The goal of yoga training is to unify body, mind, and spirit. It achieves this by co-ordination of breath and movement, mental focus, and meditation. Depending on the style of yoga, it calls for the holding of specific postures for a certain period of time, powerful movement sequencing, perfect alignment and control of the body, and flowing from one pose to another. Many of the conventional benefits of exercise may be achieved through yoga, such as muscular strength, flexibility, and cardio-respiratory fitness. The main aim of yoga is to restore the mind-body connection to its fundamental state of well-being, ease, and vibrant alertness.

It is most important that a person choose an exercise program that is suitable and safe and that resonates with his or her desires. If this is accomplished, the individual will comply with the exercise over the long term, and the activity will become his or her preferred sport. Progressing from an exercise regimen to hydrotherapy, water aerobics, Pilates, tai chi, or yoga assists the patient in moving away from a patient-oriented environment into an athletic activity and an environment that promotes health.

There are many styles of exercise that can achieve these goals. The most important aspects of exercise are that it be safe, comfortable, and enjoyable, and not increase pain. If discomfort increases minimally during exercise and then resolves, this is usually a safe style of exercise, and progress can and will be made. Since so many patients suffer from pain and feel utter and complete frustration as a result, it is important to realize that although achieving a life less dominated by pain takes time, progress can be made through exercise, the setting of meaningful and interesting goals, pacing oneself, improved coping, increasing confidence, and the knowledge that this achievement comes directly from one's own efforts.

◆ ◆ ◆

The following is a case study that may bring hope to many patients who have had failed back surgeries.

CASE STUDY

Female, age forty-six, with failed back syndrome after six surgeries to the spine.

The patient had severe back pain and was unable to work or perform normal activities of daily living.

In 1994, when I was very healthy and fit, I was involved in a motor vehicle accident, as a result of which my spine was injured. I subsequently had to leave a career that I loved very much—I was a medical representative—and I have not worked since.

Through a series of errors on the part of my doctors, I ended up having six spinal operations, two of which were through the anterior route, which is very painful, as the incision is made through the abdomen and diaphragm. I had many plates and screws in my spine, which were removed during the last two operations.

I was in the hospital for weeks at a time, feeling very depressed and lonely, as my friends visited less and less often. I vividly remember one operation when a lot of plates and screws were inserted. As a result of an oversight, I received no morphine or pain medication in the operating room, nor for the first ten hours in intensive care. My ICU nurse had not read my file properly. The doctor had deviated for some reason from his normal protocol and had not administered morphine in surgery as usual, but I should have received it as soon as I arrived in intensive care. The nurse refused to phone the doctor in the middle of the night. By the time morphine was administered, it was too late—I was a hysterical, pathetic, weeping, embarrassed wreck. Nothing could break the pain. Something died inside me that day. My pain threshold was definitely lowered for quite a few years—I could hardly bear to visit the dentist or have my eyebrows plucked! About a month after this episode, it was discovered that the metal fixation in my spine had become undone—hence more operations!

Consequently, I was always in a lot of pain. I was considered a "difficult" patient and not treated very kindly by most of the staff. Even my surgeon told me on his rounds one morning not to make so many demands on his staff! I felt trapped by all the tubes and machines, and I felt abused at the same time. I was treated as "just a spine," not like a whole human being. I was extremely depressed.

I took my rehabilitation very seriously, taking exercise classes, going for physiotherapy every week, and walking at least an hour a day. The pain became bearable at times, but I was never without pain and had to take anti-inflammatories continuously. I understood that all I could hope for as I grew older was not to deteriorate very much fur-

ther in terms of pain. Well, I was determined not to deteriorate! The specialist also envisioned a possibility of two operations in the future, one on my spine and one on my neck. I was determined to postpone these surgeries as long as possible.

About two years ago, I started going for treatment of a complementary nature: a combination of physiotherapy, electrotherapy, and acupuncture. The therapist told me that I could expect an improvement in the pain and mobility, that I would eventually only visit her once a month, and that I would be able to wean myself off the anti-inflammatories! Taken my history, it was hard to believe her, but I decided to be very positive. I had nothing to lose! She encouraged good back hygiene (I will not do anything that might compromise my spine—it is just not worth it), correct posture, exercises, and a more positive state of mind. In short, I had to change my lifestyle and outlook. She empathized so much with my pain and the bad experiences I had endured. She treated me like a whole human being and not "just a spine." This was like a breath of fresh air and changed me for the better.

As my treatments progressed, the thought that I could improve began to sink in. I believed that I would surprise everyone—that I would lead a normal life, that I would sometimes be pain-free without medication, and that I would be much more mobile. This time I was determined not only to stop the possible deterioration, but also to actually get better, to get well again, to have more mobility—definitely no more operations! That belief was the core of my healing process. I participated in water aerobics, Pilates, and other holistic treatments at the physiotherapy, acupuncture, and rehabilitation center. I read widely, including *The Journey to Pain Relief*, on all of these subjects. I am now able to do my swimming and exercises at home and to go walking at least five days per week.

I can now stretch out my physiotherapy sessions, which include mobilization, massage, electric current, and acupuncture, to once a month, but I mostly prefer to keep my appointment every two weeks. It took a lot of patience and determination on my therapist's part and mine to get where I am now, but it was all worthwhile. I went for classes in meditation and relaxation, which I also practice every day. I realized that in order to heal my spine, I had to heal my whole body—physically, psychologically, and spiritually.

Now, most of the time I am not aware of pain and I am not taking any anti-inflammatories. I am able to do more than before, like cooking (I could not stand on my feet for very long before) and also simple things like driving and grocery shopping. I do sewing or découpage for short periods at a time, watching my posture and changing my position every so often. I also know when to stop. I can sit on any chair without discomfort (I could not go to the movies or restaurants before). I can stand in a queue. But I will not lift, push, or pull heavy objects, or do any particular activity for too long. I will not work in the garden anymore—it is just not worth it!

Yes, I am a different person from two years ago. I have my off days, but I never despair, as I know what is possible and that, eventually, I will have fewer off days. I cope 100 percent.

I encourage everybody who experiences pain not to despair. There is hope. There is a lot that can be done to alleviate the situation, not only by your therapist, but also by yourself. You have to be de-termined to get better, 24/7. You have to change your lifestyle and your outlook. This means rethinking how you live, how you think, and how you feel. I understand how you feel now—like how can anyone understand? Is there any hope? Will I need more operations? First, find the right therapist. Then, trust her, and follow her advice to the letter. I went for the operations much too quickly—I know one feels desperate and will do anything to alleviate the pain, but please go for other opinions before taking such a big step.

I make a habit of never discussing my previous or present pain or operations or spine or whatever with other people, even my close friends. When asked, I reply that I am fine. It is not their fault that they have not been where I have been, that they cannot really understand. Such discussions would also continually remind one of the pain—giving power to a negative thought. Find one person to discuss your pain with when needed—be it your spouse, a very special friend, or therapist. I choose to discuss my pain with my therapist on my visits—that is it.

I know that most of my friends have forgotten about my unfortunate accident and operations, that they see me as a healthy, fit, and very positive person, and as somebody who has done a lot of internal growing, and still does! I have also surprised quite a few radiologists and other specialists who find it hard to believe that I am so very, very well, given what my X rays reveal. Which shows you, it's only X rays—a spine—and remember, you are a whole human being.

CHAPTER 12

COPING SKILLS

C hronic-pain patients are often presented with two challenges: how to prevent pain, and, perhaps even more difficult, how to cope once pain attacks.

Every chronic-pain patient has to prepare for the eventuality of pain. Many patients live with and alongside pain. If methods are not found to counter or alleviate maximal pain, their quality of life severely deteriorates, and some of them cannot continue with their lives as they knew them.

Frida, a film about the Mexican artist Frida Kahlo, who lived in the 1920s, reveals the intense suffering that pain can cause. As a teenager, Kahlo sustained severe injuries to her spine and pelvis from a bus accident. She endured constant and severe pain. At one point she exclaimed, "Pain changes you!"

Being prepared for pain and armed with countermeasures empowers the patient and relieves the fear of pain, anxiety, stress, and/ or disability. This chapter is full of such countermeasures: helpful tips for any painful condition. We all have favorite procedures or treatments that we have tried and tested and have found successful for our own particular conditions. I hope this chapter offers you some suggestions that you have not tried. Perhaps one or more of them will be of value in *your* situation.

Keep a Progress Diary

Keeping a diary will help you to evaluate the day's activities. It will illustrate those activities that created irritation or disturbance of the painful condition, as well as those that enhanced your day.

If an activity disturbed the day, such as shopping, that activity does not have to be completely avoided, but you may wish to restrict it in terms of duration and effort. Consider asking a friend to help. At the same time, it is important to at least perform the activity and achieve success, even if only in a small way. This is called pacing yourself.

Example: If doing the whole household shopping caused pain, divide the shopping list into three or four smaller and shorter trips. Make sure to wear supportive shoes and a neck or back brace, and to use a walker or crutch, if necessary, both when doing the shopping and unloading the groceries. Remember to make use of the grocery cart as a support.

Important: After the strenuous activity, rest on the bed or sit in a comfortable chair and read, watch your favorite television program, and/or have a cup of something enjoyable, preferably nonalcoholic, for twenty minutes before progressing with other activities. This rest can make all the difference in the pain level for the rest of the day.

Meditate

Resting for at least twenty or thirty minutes a day is good for everyone. It activates the parasympathetic nervous system, relaxes the sympathetic nervous system, heals the body, and rests brain activity.

Consider practicing what is known as mindfulness meditation before resting. (It may be helpful to take a meditation class to find a form of meditation that works for you.) Mindfulness meditation achieves a mind that is calm and stable. The meditator has to reach a conscious and mindful state, which requires practice and focus. Mindfulness meditation is practiced universally, has no relationship to any religion, and is used by psychologists and in pain clinics to assist patients to relax and ease pain. Focus your mind on peaceful thoughts, allowing

nothing to disturb or distress you. Let your thoughts drift away, and remain in a peaceful and calm frame of mind. It is important to remember that, once the mind is calm, thoughts may arise. Acknowledge them, and then let them pass easily, without becoming disturbed by them. Use a word, a sound, an object, or a phrase that allows you to focus your mind to achieve peacefulness. Visualization and breathing exercises will also predispose you to a meditative state. Once you have become accustomed to this peaceful state of mind, this technique may be used when a stressful occasion arises, when you feel angry or disturbed by an event, or when you have pain. Practice this meditative state for at least twenty minutes at a time, preferably daily.

According to a report in *The New York Times,* recent studies by Dr. R. Davidson, director of the Laboratory for Affective Neuroscience on fMRI (functional MRI), at the University of Wisconsin, revealed that when patients are anxious, angry, and depressed, both the amygdala, a part of the brain's emotional center, and the right prefrontal cortex are activated. When patients feel upbeat, enthusiastic, and energized, those sites are quiet and there is more activity in the left prefrontal cortex.[1] The right prefrontal area is important for hypervigilance and is typically active in people under stress. It has been hypothesized that mindfulness meditation may strengthen an array of neurons in the left prefrontal cortex that inhibit (block) the messages from the amygdala that drive disturbing emotions.[2] Using mindfulness meditation, people learn to monitor their moods and thoughts and to drop those that might spin them toward distress.

In an article published in the *Journal of Psychosomatic Medicine,* also mentioned in *The New York Times,* Davidson and John Kabat-Zinn, founders of the Mindfulness-Based Stress Reduction Clinic, at the University of Massachusetts Medical School, in Worcester, report that giving workers training in mindfulness meditation[3]

◆ reduces activity in the stress areas of the brain

◆ improves mood

◆ increases energy

◆ decreases anxiety

◆ improves work concentration

◆ improves the strength of the immune system

Practicing these meditative techniques may have profound effects on the left side of the brain, strengthening neurons and benefiting the general health of the pain sufferer.

Exercise

If you are very weak and unfit and have only been able to lie down most of the time, start somewhere to become more active:

◆ Sit in a chair for twenty or thirty minutes daily, then do so two to three times a day.

◆ If possible, move the joints that are not painful, such as the feet, ankles, knees, hips, hands, wrists, elbows, shoulders, and neck. Move every joint five to ten times.

If you are unfit and have not been moving around much, you need some exercise. Start walking to the end of your yard, the end of the building, or the end of the block on which you live—whatever you think you can manage.

◆ Time yourself and try to return in a shorter time period each time in order to build up your aerobic capacity.

◆ Stay at this level for at least three days to one week, and then start to increase the distance that you walk.

◆ Walking twenty to thirty minutes every day will increase your fitness and aerobic capacity and will also calm and focus the mind. Concentrating on an activity is also a form of mindfulness meditation.

◆ Make a plan to move every hour at work. Get up, stretch, and walk about, even if it is only to get a glass of water.

◆ Plan to include an exercise program in your life—visit the gym, join an exercise class, ride a bicycle, swim, or join a walking club.

◆ Exercise at least three times a week, and work up to five times a week, if possible.

◆ Do not plan a strenuous exercise every day of the week; give yourself a little time to rest your body in between routines.

◆ Give yourself *time for yourself!*

If you're homebound or bed-bound:

◆ Move every part of your body that you can possibly move and that is not involved in the pain.

◆ Repeat every few hours.

◆ Try to move the painful region, unless there is an unstabilized fracture or profound disease process.

- Exercise in your warm bath.
- Experience a hydrotherapy session in a heated pool.
- Try to exercise in a heated pool.

Remember: If you don't use it, you lose it!

Medicate as Needed

Medication may be necessary to improve your activity and to cope with life skills and pain levels. Take medication as prescribed by your doctor. When you begin to feel a little better, consider discussing with your doctor the following methods of reducing your use of anti-inflammatories and painkillers:

- Take half a tablet instead of a full tablet daily
- Take one tablet three or four times a week
- Possibly take an extra tablet (on consultation with the doctor) before certain difficult chores or exercise regimens

Use TENS

Perhaps you have tried a TENS unit and there was no pain relief. I suggest you try TENS according to the following method before discarding it as a useless mechanism for you (see also Appendix B):

- Place the negative electrode (which has a black connection on the wire lead) on the most painful site.
- Place the positive electrode (which has a red connection on the wire lead) either above, on the side of, or below the painful site—whatever seems practical. (See

Appendix B for diagrams recommending placement of TENS electrodes.)

- The diagrams for the MDC electrode placements may also be helpful (Appendix C), except that the MDC electrodes need to be widely spaced (four electrodes apart), while the TENS electrodes of opposite polarity may be placed next to one another (but not touching one another).

Set the controls as follows:

- Select the highest frequency or rate of pulses possible on your device, at a suggested level of 200 Hz (rate of pulses).
- Choose a width of 80 milliseconds for the pulse.
- Choose a *modulation mode* instead of burst or constant.
- Adjust the intensity until you definitely feel the pins and needles as a comfortable stroking sensation, because a non-sensation will not help at all.

Try to leave the TENS in the area of the pain for at least eight hours a day for three days. Continue with all your normal activities while using the TENS, but do not sleep with the TENS unit as it may disturb your sleep or the electrodes may move during the night and produce an unpleasant sensation.

As previously mentioned, you may have complete resolution of your pain within three days, or you may find that you are greatly eased by the TENS and the actual pain level itself becomes more tolerable.

It is suggested that you use TENS while undertaking difficult tasks or while participating in sports that experience has shown will increase your pain. Continue with the TENS for at least forty minutes after you have completed the difficult task or sports activity.

If you require TENS to control your pain levels, use it at least once a day for forty minutes. There is no overdosage with TENS. You may, however, adapt to the current, making it necessary to increase the intensity as the current becomes less noticeable.

You may also become tolerant to the endogenous opioids released by the TENS treatment. This means that, after three days of treatment, the TENS effect may not retain its efficacy in some individuals. This problem can be solved by stopping treatment after three days and then resuming two or three days later. Continue treating in this manner if you have this response to TENS treatment.

You may use the TENS on different areas at the same time, as there are usually two lead wires with a negative and a positive attached to each one.

Do not become lazy or afraid to reach for your TENS unit for pain relief. It may become the best friend you ever had!

Make Use of the "Electrical Anti-Inflammatory"

Direct current (MDC) is known for its anti-inflammatory, regenerative, and pain-relieving properties. It is not as universally obtainable as the TENS devices are, however.

The following are suggestions for MDC use (see also Appendix C):

◆ It is only necessary to use it for short periods—four, eight, or sixteen minutes, depending on the instructions attached to the specific device—typically once a day (but it can be applied twice a day).

◆ It can be used both to treat a specific problem when it occurs and to prevent problems from occurring.

◆ It can be used once a day as a regenerative, energizing health treatment, and it can be part of your armamentarium of treatments for your particular condition.

◆ Use according to the instructions provided in the information booklet that comes with your particular device.

Try Electrodermal Patches

New technology has developed electrodermal (skin) patches that release a slight, often unnoticeable microelectric current. This treatment is especially recommended for patients with severe pain who are sensitive to touch. The effect is gentle stimulation of the tissue and activation of the body's natural healing processes with no side effects.

Apply Heat or Cold

Both heat and cold may be useful. They should be used on a test basis to see which of the two helps the most with your particular problem. Heat may help with low-back pain, but not with a painful and inflamed ankle. Try each one to prove its suitability for the particular condition.

Both modalities relieve pain and inflammation and improve circulation. General rules for the application of heat or cold are as follows:

◆ When a joint is hot and/or swollen, use ice to decrease the heat and the swelling.

- When a joint aches, especially in cold weather, use heat.
- Apply either of these treatments when discomfort arises.
- Apply both of these treatments sequentially, if appropriate, especially with swelling, to improve the circulation.
- Use for at least twenty minutes.

Many people prefer heat, as it is more comfortable and easier to apply. Heat can be provided by the following:

- A simple hot-water bottle
- A heated electrical pad
- A bag (usually with special seeds) that is microwaveable
- A bag of specialized gel that can be placed in boiling water to increase and maintain heat
- A hot pack (may contain mud—a sandy substance that retains heat)

Caution: When applying heat, always use towels or other fabric to protect the skin and prevent skin burns.

Cold or ice can be provided by the following:

- A bag of frozen peas or other vegetables (not particularly hygienic!)
- A bag of ice cubes
- A bag of specialized gel that can be placed in the freezer
- A cold, medicated spray

Here's the best, most comfortable, and safest method of applying ice:

- Place a wet, warm towel around or on the painful site.
- Place the ice pack over the towel on the painful site. This allows the area to accommodate the cold more gently.

Use these modalities when discomfort arises. It is amazing how a simple procedure such as heat or ice can relieve pain or discomfort.

Get a Massage

Therapeutic touch or massage is beneficial for pain, due to the fact that the pain-relief receptors are being stimulated.

Rules:

- If massage helps, then rub away!
- Rub or gently hold the painful area.
- Deep massage or pressure on trigger points can relieve muscle spasm.
- If massage irritates, do not use this modality.

Try Acutouch

Some patients are able to purchase their own acutouch device (see Chapter 4), which can be used daily as a preventive and healing procedure, or whenever pain and inflammation occur. Acutouch is a device that activates and stimulates healing at acupuncture points and may relieve pain and inflammation in any external area of the body. It produces a biological current that is said to affect the electrical polarity and energetic activity in acupuncture points and body tissues, enhancing the immune system. It uses a combination of microelectric current, magnetic fields, and a special lens that focuses light waves with no external electrical source.

Apply Topical Medications

Rubbing various preparations onto the skin may be extremely helpful for pain and inflammation. It is wonderful to be able to help yourself from the outside (by using a cream or other preparation) and also to help yourself on the inside by using a beneficial medication. Using these applications simultaneously reduces pain levels, allowing you to cope much better!

There are many brands of anti-inflammatory creams, both herbal and allopathic, on the market. You may find that applying a cream and then placing the hot-water bottle or ice pack over the area increases the effect of the medication due to improved circulation.

Anti-inflammatory dermal patches are available that may be applied to the pain site for a specific period of time. Your doctor may also prescribe patches with stronger medications, such as morphine, usually to be applied daily. These may be applied anywhere on the body (not necessarily on the painful site).

New creams have been developed, such as those made from capsicum, which is derived from the hot chili pepper. This substance is inexpensive and highly effective in relieving pain; it has the advantage of dredging substance P from the tissues to which it is applied. Substance P increases pain; when it is removed from the tissues (skin, soft tissues, spinal cord, or brain), pain is relieved. Capsicum can only be applied to the skin and may not reach higher nervous centers.

It is best to use a combination of capsicum and aloe vera or another soothing substance; capsicum by itself may produce an intolerable burning sensation. A small amount may be applied three times a day on a painful area. Over a period of time, pain levels will be reduced. It should not be used only as needed, but as a specific regimen over a specific period of time.

There are many different preparations available; you need to investigate and find the one(s) that will most help you.

Herbal Remedies

Herbal oils, mixed in carrier creams, are used to reduce inflammation and pain. They may also be used in the bath for rest, destressing, and relaxation. Many people prefer to burn them in a burner and utilize the fragrance for relaxation, antianxiety effects, and improvement of sleep.

S. Ruegg, a Swiss medical technologist with expertise in herbal medicine, has developed healing creams with powerful medicinal effects and has suggested the remedies below for the relief of various types of pain and discomfort.[4]

HERBS AND OILS TO ADD TO A CREAM BASE FOR ARTHRITIS	
Comfrey	Aids in mending fractures
Lavender	Pain-relieving and antirheumatic
Basil essential oil	Healing and calming
Devil's claw tincture	Anti-inflammatory

HERBS AND OILS TO ADD TO A CREAM BASE FOR NERVE PAIN, SUCH AS IN CRPS OR INFLAMED NERVE ENDINGS	
St. John's wort infused in olive oil	Antidepressant and stimulates regeneration of nerves
Organic lavender, lavender essential oil	Pain-relieving and antibacterial
Organic basil, basil essential oil	Healing and calming

HERBS FOR DRINKING IN A TEA	
Chamomile	Anti-inflammatory, calming and soothing
Rosemary	Improves the circulation (not for patients with high blood pressure, except in cooking)
Ginger	Pain-relieving, antioxidant

Try Magnets

As discussed in Chapter 4, using small magnets over a particularly painful area may help relieve pain and improve mobility. You can immediately test the benefit of the small magnet(s) by performing a previously painful movement to see if the magnet helps your pain or stiffness.

Tips for using magnets:

◆ Move the magnets around on the painful area to achieve maximum benefit.

◆ Place the negative pole on the pain site.

◆ Magnets are most effective over the pain.

◆ Use a magnet continuously for at least five days for maximum benefit.

◆ Rest for two days.

◆ Reapply, if necessary.

◆ Magnets should last indefinitely.

◆ If the magnet increases the pain, remove it.

There are many types of magnetic braces for any area of the body, and even magnetic blankets and bedding. You will never know how successful magnets may be unless you try them!

Perform Breathing Exercises

We all breathe all the time, whether we want to or not, but it is the quality of the breath that is important. Most people breathe using shallow breaths. This limits oxygenation in the body, decreases healing, and does not help pain.

Here is how to breathe beneficially:

◆ Take the time to lie or sit in a relaxed and comfortable position.

◆ Place both hands, with fingers touching, on the stomach, just below the rib cage.

◆ Place the tongue behind the back of the front upper teeth; this relaxes the jaw and the neck muscles.

◆ Take a deep breath in through the nose, allowing the area under the hands on the stomach to lift or swell as the lungs expand. Try to count silently to five as you inhale.

◆ Close the eyes and feel the lungs filling up with oxygen and air.

- Feel the whole rib cage expanding as you breathe in. Allow the air to reach down as far as your lower back.

- Hold the breath in for four or five counts.

- Slowly exhale and allow the hands to sink down as you breathe out.

- Breathe out through the nose, if possible, trying to count to five. If you breathe out through the mouth, the tongue loses its position behind the back of the front teeth.

- If you cannot hold your breath for as long as five counts, then count to whatever number is comfortable for you. Try to increase the length of time you spend on each part of the breath: the inhale, the hold, and the exhale.

- Perform this exercise for at least ten minutes.

This procedure may be used daily as relaxation training—and surprise—the pain may also be relieved. It can also be used to help minimize discomfort when you do have pain, or when you are about to experience a procedure that may become uncomfortable, such as a visit to the dentist.

Visualize

Take your thoughts on a holiday. Closing the eyes and visualizing a wonderful place that you find especially relaxing, soothing, and enjoyable is almost the same as being there.

There are many forms of visualization. Here are some suggestions:

A journey using the colors of the rainbow

- Start with breathing exercises and some peaceful music that you enjoy.

- Imagine that you are walking on a mountain path. You come across a field of brilliant red poppies with tiny black centers, as far as the eye can see.

- Stand still and just take it all in.

- Continue on, and enter an orange grove where oranges are hanging from the trees. The oranges look so beautiful against the green of the leaves, and you can smell the wonderful citrus aroma drifting toward you.

- Take your time and walk slowly through the grove.

- As you move along the path and start to climb the mountain, you can see a patch of sunflowers as you look down on the other side of the valley below, so bright that all you can see is a splash of yellow.

- There is a wonderful smell of greenery and grass as you relax and gaze down on this scene.

- Next, you enter a forested area where it feels cool and moist under your feet. There is a canopy of green above and all around you.

- As you wander through the forest, you pass little streams with rocks at the edges of the pools. Sit down and put your feet in the cool water. Listen to the water as it falls over the rocks.

- As you come out of the forest, you notice that the sky is so blue that it almost takes your breath away. Rest against a tree, and just enjoy the deep blue of the sky. It eventually fades into a warm, pinky glow, and then to a soft, velvety purple.

There are many other examples that may resonate with you:

- Imagine taking a walk along a desert island with the sea crashing on the sand.
- Visualize yourself sitting on a rock looking out to sea and hearing the waves crash along the seashore.

Only you will know what makes you feel wonderful!

In addition, research demonstrates successful ways of changing the pain experience by changing the way that you think about the pain in terms of words, color, size, shape, and any other manner in which pain might represent itself to you.[5] Here's how: Guide yourself into a state of relaxation by closing your eyes and breathing deep, allowing yourself to be revitalized by each breath and feeling more peaceful. Expand your inner space, becoming alert, quiet, and watchful, yet detached.

Now describe your pain in silence to yourself. Be present with the pain; know that the pain may be either physical sensations or worries or fears or anything—whatever comes into your mind. Let the pain take on a shape, size, color, texture, sound.

Now, with your eyes still closed, cup your palms together, and put the pain object in your hand. How would you change it (size, color, texture, sound)? There's no right or wrong way to finish the experience; just ac-

cept what feels right to you. Throw the pain away or place it where you found it or move it to somewhere else. As you do, let yourself become aware of how pain can change.

You may be surprised to find that as you intentionally modify the pain in your thoughts, the pain will physically change and become more acceptable and manageable.

Here's another technique: Close your eyes, and imagine your painful site (e.g., your swollen, stiff, and painful knee) in your mind's eye. Now imagine *this:*

- The swelling is reducing and the knee is getting thinner—you can now fit into your trousers.
- The pain is fading away, first from one area and then another.
- The painful area is becoming smaller and smaller.
- You can now move the knee with ease in a range that was previously impossible.
- You can visualize yourself effortlessly riding a stationary bicycle.
- You are taking a ride down the road on your bicycle.
- Now you are enjoying a brisk walk or a run down a lovely shady road. Remain in this visualization for at least five minutes, or as long as you are comfortable with these thoughts.

Here are the tricks to make visualization work for you:

- Think clearly and carefully.
- Do not allow emotions to enter your mind.

- If you have a thought that distracts you, just let it go.
- Think, "I am going to heal. My bone will knit, my knee will bend, my pain will go!"

This calm, clear, and precise attitude actually helps the visualization exercise be more effective by triggering the body to release substances that stimulate healing and pain relief. By contrast, once emotions arise that interfere with clear thoughts, anxiety and stress may disturb the mind and limit healing. Substances are then released that hamper or block the natural healing process.

Practice Self-Hypnosis

Self-hypnosis is the ability to alter physical symptoms by making suggestions to the conscious mind. This safe and controllable exercise is a powerful tool to enable you to create endorphins in the brain that descend to the painful areas of the body. A hypnotic experience is consciously induced. You can start with therapeutic suggestions given to you by your therapist.

Self-hypnosis is a skill that takes practice. Once learned, it eventually assists or improves pain control. Here is a program that you can practice:

- Sit back, relax your body, get comfortable, and relax your mind. Place your tongue behind the back of the front teeth. Take a deep breath. Breathe in through your nose and out through your nose or mouth. Picture a favorite scene, place, or activity.

- Breathe in for four counts, hold for four counts, and breathe out for four counts. Let nothing disturb or bother you; allow your thoughts to roam in and out of your consciousness without any undue concern about their meaning or content. It would not surprise me if you notice some change now, as the body feels more relaxed and you become more comfortable with yourself.
- Just concentrate on breathing: in, hold, out.
- A warm, heavy, relaxed, numb, or tired feeling may come over you after a while. Perhaps transfer this feeling to the back, neck, or wherever you hurt.
- Thoughts may begin to come into your mind that are emotional; tears may fall. The thoughts may surprise you because they may be very old memories that are rising to the surface to be acknowledged, accepted, and released.
- Let the warm, heavy, relaxed, numb, tired feeling continue to wash over you. It may even be possible that this pleasant feeling will continue after the session. You may be surprised to find that you can easily achieve this feeling yourself when you're alone. This is your very own achievement.
- You may be pleasantly surprised to find that the pain has diminished, is less noticeable, and becomes more manageable. You may find that you have developed another method of pain control and that you have managed to achieve some comfortable relaxation time.

Remember that you are entitled to have time for yourself to improve your own health!

◆ Before opening your eyes, count down from four to one, and know that you are going to feel relaxed and refreshed and can more easily cope with your pain.

Relax

Some people need to feel their muscles tense before they can relax them. The body and brain may need to recognize the difference between a tense and a relaxed muscle. Use the following relaxation suggestions:

◆ Relax in a comfortable position, sitting or lying, but avoid the temptation of falling asleep.

◆ Use the breathing exercise as outlined above.

◆ Starting with the toes, and working your way up to the top of your head, tighten each group of muscles, hold for three seconds, and then release completely. Tighten and then release your toes, calf muscles, thighs, buttocks, stomach and back muscles, fingers, wrists, arms, shoulders, and facial muscles.

◆ If you are not yet relaxed, repeat once or twice until the body feels completely relaxed.

◆ When you are finally feeling fully re-laxed, sit or lie in this position, using visualization and/or breathing to aug-ment the relaxation, for at least ten to twenty minutes.

Observe Good Posture and Ergonomics

Always try to maintain good posture what-ever the activity you are engaged in, whether work, recreation, or relaxation.

Here are pointers for maintaining good posture while you are at work:

◆ Sit at a desk that allows you to retain a comfortable posture. Use a cushion, if necessary, to support the spine or a stool to lift the feet. If you spend hours at the computer, be sure you have your work area set up ergonomically (see "Tips for Sitting at a Desk," in Chapter 3).

◆ If you constantly use the telephone, use a headpiece to prevent irritation to the neck, which happens when one persis-tently maintains the head in a tilted position.

◆ Keep the back straight, and use the ab-dominal muscles and the knees when bending to pick up articles.

◆ Hold and lift heavy parcels close to the body.

◆ Use a cervical collar or back brace dur-ing exertion or difficult activities, but remove the collar or brace when doing easier chores.

◆ Use a cervical collar for driving if doing so is comfortable and if wearing one allows you to see the road properly.

◆ If you have an occupation that requires much standing, arrange to have a thick rubber mat or carpet to stand on. A mat or carpet cushions weight bear-ing, reduces pressure on the spine, and relieves tension in all the muscles of the body.

Most people experience pain at work or during leisure activities because they retain positions for long periods and their posture is not perfect. When the posture is correct, many muscles are working to hold you in an upright position. Your best exercise when remaining still or holding a position for any length of time is to work or exercise the muscle-support system by actively observing good posture.

Recognize the Importance of Sleep

Sleep is when the body repairs itself. It is a necessary part of life. Certain endogenous chemicals, such as serotonin, are necessary to promote sleep. Some patients who suffer from fibromyalgia and other conditions (e.g., anxiety, obsessive-compulsive disorder, bulimia, excess body weight, restless-leg syndrome, and tension or migraine headaches) have low levels of serotonin. This decreases the quality of their sleep, diminishes their recuperative period, and increases their pain levels.

Pain can be so severe that it interferes with sleep, impacting negatively on healing and pain relief. Patients may often feel so exhausted that they fall asleep too early, which in turn produces wakefulness at inappropriate times and feeds the cycle of exhaustion and sleeplessness. The body has a circadian rhythm that affects levels of hormones and other substances; if this rhythm is disturbed, it impacts on metabolic processes and ultimately affects health.

Here are some tips for getting a good night's sleep:

◆ It is useful to have a rest during the day (at midday) to enable oneself to fall asleep at appropriate times.

◆ Try to exercise each day to attain a naturally tired state.

◆ Before going to sleep at night, read something boring.

◆ Take recommended pain relievers before sleep, if pain disturbs your sleep.

◆ Drink an herbal tea without caffeine, such as chamomile, before retiring.

◆ Place lavender drops on the pillow before sleeping (be sure to avoid eye contact).

◆ Take a warm bath in water laced with lavender and other soothing preparations to improve relaxation before going to sleep.

◆ If you have a bladder problem, drinking should be avoided or minimized after 6:00 P.M.

◆ If the room is too cold:
  – Dress warmly
  – Use sufficient blankets on the bed
  – Use a covered and secured hot-water bottle in the bed
  – Use a small heater in the room

◆ If the room is too hot:
  – Keep the windows open
  – Use lighter bed linen or merely a sheet to cover the body
  – Use a fan—preferably overhead

Set Goals and Pace Yourself

- Make all your goals realistic.

- Perform an activity that is possible.

- Do not try to do the impossible.

- Do not *overdo* activities that *are* possible.

- Plan your day, but be prepared for the unexpected.

- Plan to do something each day that is helpful, that encourages exercise, and that makes progress in your condition and in your life.

As previously mentioned, it is not helpful to increase activity so much that afterward your pain and your condition regress. Having a goal and reaching it is a great achievement, and only *you* can do this for yourself.

◆ ◆ ◆

You are now armed with suggestions and activities that may help to remove some of the obstacles in the path to pain relief. There are many different ways to improve matters. You may have discovered certain treatments or plans to encourage you when a flare-up occurs, and you may now be more prepared to help yourself improve.

Bear the following in mind:

- Implementing these applications requires effort and thought.

- Make the effort, and do not become disturbed because the pain is still with you.

- Do not expect the pain to go away until, through your efforts, it eventu-

ally disappears or becomes much less noticeable.

- Make this task your own journey of discovery, and you will soon achieve a satisfactory result.

CASE STUDY

A fifty-seven-year-old female who had undergone a total knee replacement and suffered severe knee and leg pain, swelling in the knee, stiffness, and an inability to walk without crutches.

Chronic pain itself is my disease. My knee now works after seven days a week of treatment at a pain and rehabilitation clinic. My treatment combines Western and Eastern techniques to relieve the swelling and allow the knee to bend naturally. The joint works but the pain remains.

After two years of living hourly with this pain, I am not who I used to be, except some of the time, and then there are moments of euphoria and I glow again and people around me laugh at my subtlety and wit. But it does not happen often. I always had masses of energy and needed very little sleep, but now when I'm cooking, the pots weigh so much, and short, abrupt turning movements seem to hurt the most; my knee feels like it is made out of wood and barbed wire, with "boiling iced water" being thrown at me like knife slashes.

It's hard not to show the pain. At some point I realize I have been hiding it for hours and the one extra inconvenience in my day makes me burst! I get so ashamed. My beloved partner thinks that I don't want to entertain. I become sly at finding moments to put my leg up, and I pace myself all day. I hear myself say that I have become a cripple, and nobody contradicts me. I am in danger of becoming a bore!

I am totally subjective about this pain. It's not only the physical aspect (although it has taken many months to cease trying to find a physical answer). It's what it does: the anxiety about every occasion that gnaws in secrecy at my spirit, the loneliness of hiding it that spreads like a desert. Pain overthrows my spirit—it is an unpleasant, draining emotional experience, a constant stress on my mind and body and behavior.

Today, I took painkillers. I don't often. When my hair started falling out from these drugs, I realized that no doctor was going to control this unseen monster stalking me in my shadow. I had to. Medication does not change what I think, or feel, or do. My behavior and the reaction to me of those I love depend on self-awareness and a really effective, quality, close relationship. Water aerobics, my posture, good nutrition, stretching, pacing myself, and taking an ongoing interest in a much bigger world beyond myself are all ingredients in coping. Keeping a mental diary has helped a lot. Last year I could not turn on the hose at the side of the garden—not even when using two crutches.

I can live a productive and constructive life with my chronic pain. I will learn to manage this pain by using my brain, my body, and my psyche.

The journey to pain relief is a great adventure for you. Once you succeed, your personal happiness and growth will know no bounds.

ACUPUNCTURE TECHNIQUES FOR SPECIFIC CONDITIONS

According to S. Peilin, the traditional Chinese medicine (TCM) approach to pain management "treats the cause of the problem (mostly stagnation of Qi and blood), promotes the Qi and blood circulation, calms the mind[,] and regulates the heart to diminish pain and prevent recurrences."[1] This section of the book is for therapists and clinicians who practice acupuncture in general and for those who treat pain, especially chronic pain, in particular. As far as I know, no specific acupuncture guidelines or treatments have been published for the pain clinic or the chronic-pain patient. The future of chronic-pain treatment will be enhanced by ongoing understanding and development of a biomedical acupuncture model that incorporates both the traditional Chinese and the Western scientific approaches. Our responsibility to chronic-pain patients is to increase our knowledge of scientifically proven information and to expand our armamentarium to improve pain relief.

The acupuncture points and techniques described below are recommended for treating different types of pain and its ramifications (depression, anxiety) in various conditions. The recommended protocols originate from a wide variety of sources and have been clinically tested and proven by the author. They have helped many patients.

Instructions for All Acupuncture Treatments, Unless Otherwise Indicated

All points indicated on the diagrams in this Appendix provide the general position of the acupoints. Only persons qualified and knowledgeable in acupuncture should attempt to locate and insert needles into the points. There are many acupuncture books and atlases that indicate the correct positioning of these points.

All points are used bilaterally, where appropriate.

Points may be added that include all the areas relevant to the treatment of the pain. Select all other relevant additional points that relate to the condition and the pain. Add distal points in scalp, ears, or limbs, when appropriate, to increase pain relief.

Points used depend upon the positioning of the patient.

Guidelines about positioning:

◆ If prone, support the lower abdomen on a pillow, and insert another pillow under the shins to flex the knees and release the lower back.

◆ If supine, support the head with one or two pillows, and position one or two pillows under the knees to relax the low back.

Duration of the treatment also depends upon the positioning of the patient:

◆ Prone: twenty to thirty minutes

◆ Supine: thirty to forty-five minutes

If the patient becomes restless or anxious during treatment, treat for a shorter duration (e.g., fifteen to twenty minutes) or withdraw the needles immediately.

Simultaneously add any electotherapy (e.g., TENS, MDC, microcurrent, or electroacupuncture) that may be appropriate for the condition.

1. Stress

When patients are asked what they think caused their problem, many usually say one of three things:

◆ "Stress"

◆ "Tension"

◆ "When I'm stressed or tense, my pain feels worse"

It is therefore generally preferable to undertake a regimen for dealing with stress—for example, as outlined in Chapter 3 of this book—and in addition to treat the following acupoints that will benefit both the stress and the painful condition.

Commence the treatment by placing the patient prone (face down) and needling the UB inner (physical) and outer (emotional) points, if appropriate to the condition. (UB refers to the urinary bladder lines on either side of the spinal column.) These points are located 1.5 cun and 3 cun, respectively, lateral to the interspace between two vertebrae. (A cun is the Chinese measurement of a divi-

sion on a patient's body.) According to J. Tin Yau So, a cun or division is represented by the distance between the dorsal edge of the two distal creases of the flexed middle finger of the patient's left hand (if female, measure the right hand).[2]

Lung	UB 13, 42
Heart	UB 15, 44
Liver	UB 18, 47
Spleen	UB 20, 49
Kidney	UB 23, 52

Du 14 (situated between the 7th cervical and the 1st thoracic vertebra; this point has an important influence on the immune system, with profound effects on inflammation and pain)

Treat for at least twenty minutes.

Other points that are relevant to the stress and/or anxiety may be included in both the prone and supine (face up) position.

This treatment is then followed by positioning the patient in a supine position with comfortable support for the head, neck, and low back. Treatment of the following points is recommended:

Du 20

Shishencong (S; these four extra points are situated 1 cun anterior, posterior, and bilateral to Du 20 and are included if the patient is deeply stressed)

Extra point 1 (at the midpoint between the medial ends of the eyebrows)

Ren 17 (between the breasts at the level of the 4th rib)

Li 4, H 7, Sp 6, Liv 3

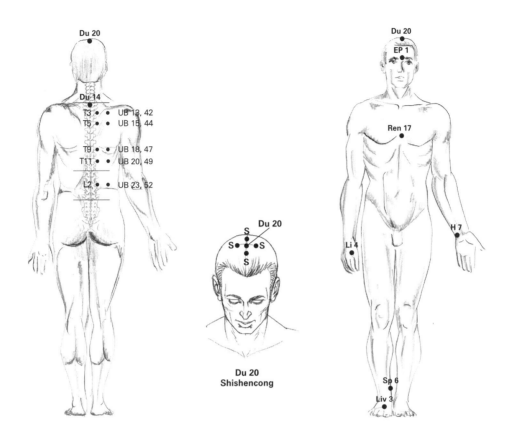

Du 20

Shishencong

H 7 treats depression, sadness, and fear, and also improves memory. Sp 6 has many powerful effects on the body but specifically calms the mind. Liv 3 treats pain, swelling, anxiety, depression, and fear.

Patients should relax in this position for at least thirty minutes.

A specific point was described by anesthetist J. Filshie at a British Medical Acupuncture Society meeting in 2003.[3] This point was initially used to treat nausea and breathlessness during chemotherapy at a cancer clinic in the United Kingdom. Not only did the protocol assist patients with their nausea and breathlessness (dysnea), but it also relieved their anxiety, sadness, and depression. Ac-

cordingly, the point was named the "anxiety, sickness, and dysnea" (ASAD) point.

Dr. Filshie's observation of patients who were receiving chemotherapy or radiation therapy, or patients who were anxious or depressed but without serious disease, demonstrated that patients were able to release their breath in the form of a large sigh shortly after insertion of a single needle to this point. Release of breath improves oxygen and circulatory supply and relieves anxiety. Changes were noted immediately after the session of treatment and maintained after only one treatment at the next session.

The point is located with a point finder centrally between Ren 17 and Ren 22 on the upper chest wall above the breasts in both sexes. When the point of lowest resistance is found, indicating the location of the ASAD point, the point finder will indicate this by emitting more sound.

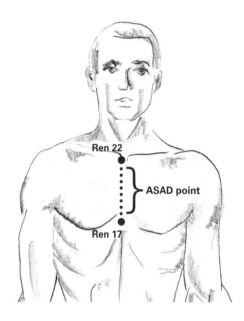

The one-needle technique allows for the needle to be left taped to the skin for at least three days. If the needle is left in this position, it must be placed very carefully so that no pain or injury will occur with any movement of the head, neck, or body.

Many patients report a feeling of relaxation and stress release following acupuncture treatment for stress. Sleep may even overwhelm them. The patient's demeanor often changes from an anxious one to a smiling and communicative one. This protocol is one of the most important aspects of any treatment for the chronic-pain patient.

2. Inflammation

An element of inflammation is present in most patients with pain. Even a small degree of inflammation may create a great deal of pain. Imagine having a boil on any area of the body. Although relatively small, it may be extremely painful. Even when the boil has healed virtually to the point of complete regression, it may still remain painful until it completely disappears. Patients often wonder why they continue to experience pain despite an evident decrease in the inflammation. Patients should be advised that until *all* inflammation has disappeared, discomfort may continue.

Suggested points for treating inflammation: Du 20, Du 14, EP 1, Li 4, Li 11, Sp 6, GB 34, Liv 3

These points appear to be similar to the aforementioned relaxation points but are used to specifically target the inflammatory process. Du 14 treats any heat or fever in the body and is a major immune point. Li 4 relieves various types of pain, reduces heat in the tissues, and reduces the body temperature when it is raised. Li 11 relieves pain in the joints (upper limbs) and back region, reduces high temperatures, and has a potent anti-inflammatory and anti-irritation effect. GB 34 relieves pain and inflammation in tendons and muscles.

Specific points that target the lumbo-sacral spine and nerve roots to produce anti-inflammatory effects in that region are as follows:

Point	Nerve root
UB 31	S1
UB 32	S2

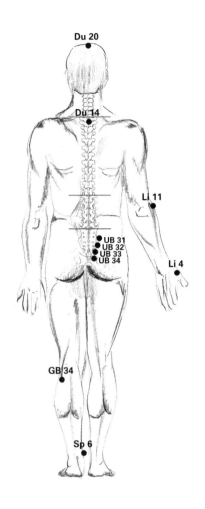

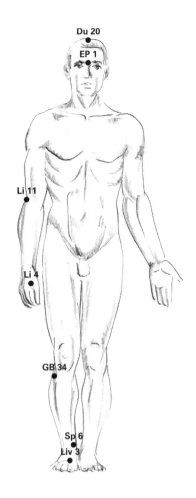

| UB 33 | S3 |
| UB 34 | S4 |

A specific protocol producing balanced levels of cortisone in the body has been advised by N. Ellis.[4] This regimen can be used with any inflammatory or hormonal disturbance that increases pain:

Bilaterally: Si 3, UB 1, UB 62

3. Immune System

As previously mentioned, the immune system works in conjunction with the opioid (pain-relieving) process.

Suggested points for treating the immune system: Du 20, Du 14, EP 1, Li 4, Li 11, St 36, Sp 6, GB 34, Liv 3

St 36 is used for treating acute abdominal pain and diseases of the anterior aspect of the lower limb, but most importantly it is

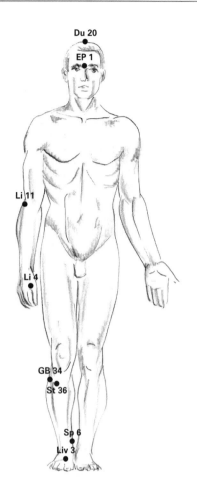
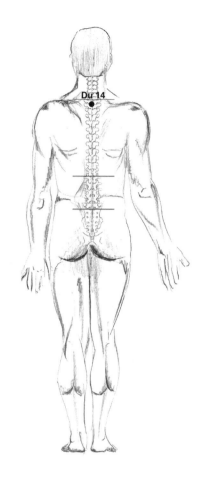

used for the prevention of disease and the promotion of good health, presumably by improving the immune system.

When the immune system functions optimally, the body is able to activate natural pain-relieving processes. It is interesting to note that if the immune system is weakened, patients cannot adequately fight infection or access optimal pain relief, as the opioid system may become deactivated or sluggish.

No system works in isolation. Therefore, each treatment should address the stress, inflammatory, and immune processes within the body, in order for healing to occur quickly

and effectively. It is notable that the medication given to patients with musculoskeletal pain usually comprises a combination of pain relievers, anti-inflammatories, muscle relaxants, antidepressants, and vitamins to relieve pain and inflammation and to protect the nervous system.

4. The Autonomic Nervous System (ANS)

St 36 and Sp 6 are known as "switches." Used in combination, they have an effect on the autonomic nervous system. According to prominent researcher and educator Dr. Linda Rapson, of Toronto, Canada, in the many protocols developed to relieve severe and sympathetically mediated pains, St 36 affects the sympathetic nervous system and Sp 6 affects the parasympathetic nervous system.[5] This combination results in the balancing of the autonomic nervous system (ANS), thus improving pain relief and good health.

Other points regarded as "switches" for the autonomic nervous system are:

Sympathetic points: Li 4, Liv 3, Du 26, Du 14, UB 23

The Du meridian is also known as the governor vessel (GV). According to the principles of traditional Chinese medicine, the governor-vessel channel can be used to strengthen the energy of the body; for example, it has a powerful influence on the spine and the kidneys. Du 26, located on the center of the philtrum, above the upper lip, affects the vasovagal system (which is responsible for fainting), calms the mind, and relieves pain. UB 23, located at the L2 (lumbar vertebra 2) treats backache, kidneys, and cold sensations in the back and limbs. Therefore, it affects circulation and the ANS. GB 20

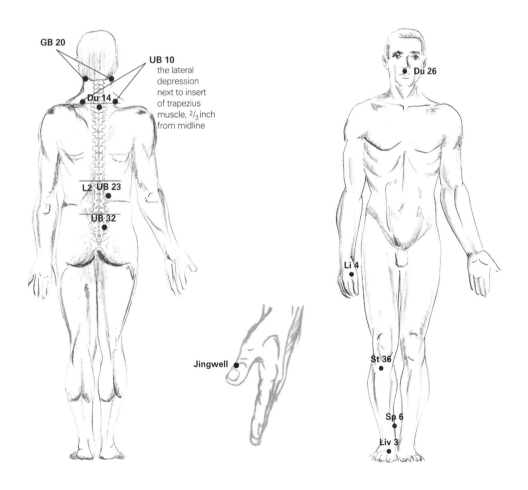

acts on the sympathetic aspect of the hypothalamus.

Parasympathetic points: H 7, UB 32, and other relevant sacral points.

UB 32 also has powerful effects on the spine and legs when treating pain and numbness. UB 10 acts on the parasympathetic aspects of the thalamus.

5. Pain

In acupuncture, pain is best addressed by treating the local area of pain, creating the "needle injury" effect, if possible. Local treatment, that is, placing needles into a painful site, may irritate the condition, but if an uncomplicated condition exists, this is the recommended approach.

It is difficult to be specific about treatment of an area that presents with pain, but the following examples may demonstrate the principles that regularly produce beneficial results.

A. Ankle Sprain

In a sprained ankle, the lateral (outside) aspect of the joint may, for example, become swollen and tender. Acupuncture needles may be inserted superficially around the swelling and into the injury.

Electrical acupuncture may be applied at a low frequency (2–4 Hz) for thirty to forty-five minutes. (Electroacupuncture is usually applied at a low frequency of between 2 and 4 Hz unless otherwise indicated.) Two or four needles will be effective locally. The efficiency of the treatment may be enhanced if distal points within the region are also used. Use the following points:

- ◆ GB 34 to activate the peroneal nerve supply to the injured region
- ◆ Liv 3 to improve pain, circulation, and mobility
- ◆ K 3 (kidney point 3) to relieve pain and improve circulation and mobility
- ◆ UB 60 to improve mobility of the whole ankle joint
- ◆ Sp 9 to improve swelling

If pain is very severe, auricular (ear) points representing the foot/ankle and pain (Shen Men) may be used initially to relieve

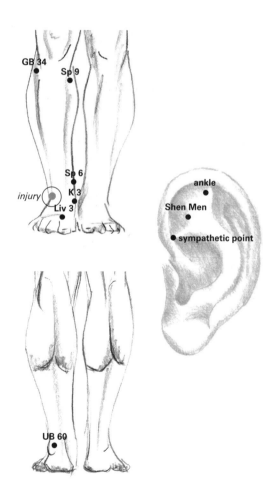

pain and improve movement. Patients are encouraged to move the affected joint once the needles have been inserted. This demonstrates to the patient that he or she has the ability to move and gain rapid pain relief. The sympathetic points in the ear are recommended if unusual symptoms are present, such as sensitivity to touch, unusual pain, temperature and circulatory (discoloration) changes, and/or swelling.

B. Back Pain

If a particular joint is painful, such as L3 and 4 (lumbar 3 and 4), insert the needles as follows:

- centrally, between the painful joints

- on each side, from L3 to L4 and from L4 to L5

- on each side of the joint (one centimeter from the spinous process—Hwa Tuo point) or one and a half *cun* (see page 158) at L3/4 and at L4/5

- electroacupuncture, applied initially to the two central needles (L3/4 and L4/5) and/or to the two needles on each side, from superior to inferior, connecting each circuit either on the right or the left of the spine but not crossing the current from the left to the right or vice versa over the spine

If muscle spasm is present around the painful joint, inserting needles deeply into the muscle spasm (IMS) will elicit a twitch response from the muscle and produce marked pain relief. The needle may be left in position for a duration of thirty seconds to one minute, or may be maintained in the same position during the above treatment for at least thirty minutes.

It is necessary to massage or use gentle pressure over the spinal and sacroiliac joints and over the lumbar, gluteal, and leg muscles to explore regions of pain and muscle spasm that are tender and that may respond to needling. Any area in the thoracic joints or muscles is related to spasm, either in the cervical (neck) or lumbar (low back) region. Treating all the areas involved in the specific patient's complaint will produce more effective results.

General and distal points may be included in the treatment of back pain, depending on the area of the pain and its referral (central, posterior, or lateral).

General points:

UB 23	one and a half *cun* from L2 (lumbar vertebra 2)
Du 4	below the spinous process of L2
UB 25	one and a half *cun* from L5
Du 3	below the spinous process of L4

Distal points:

UB 36	midpoint of the gluteal fold
UB 40	midpoint of the transverse crease of the popliteal fossa
GB 30	midway between the anterior superior border of the greater trochanter and the hiatus of the sacrum
GB 34	in the depression anterior and inferior to the small head of the fibula, near the peroneal nerve

UB 36 and 40 assist by improving spinal and hip mobility, especially increasing lumbar extension and the ability to walk. GB 30 and 34 improve back and leg pain and improve turning or rotation of the body.

If the local spinal region is severely painful, the ear points representing the spinal level involved and the sympathetic and the pain-relief points (Shen Men) are also included in the treatment.

Electric currents (discussed in Chapter 8) may also be applied to the local spinal region for pain relief.

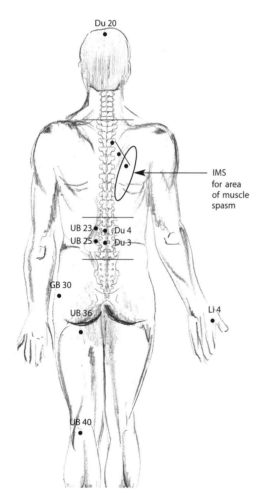

The minute needle injury that occurs in order to promote healing in a local region may irritate the tissue and nerve structures. Therefore, although probably the most effective, local treatment must be executed carefully to prevent this type of exacerbation.

Antidromic impulses are nerve impulses that travel in the opposite direction from normal nerve impulses; for example, back into the injured region. Antidromic impulses from the local nerve supplying the region (the ankle or even spinal area) may create hypersensitivity in the local and central nervous system, thus promoting swelling and excess pain that may develop into a complex regional pain syndrome. Local treatment may control this pain, or applying acupuncture to the distal points that impact the target area may then be advocated.

C. Knee Pain

The knee is a weight-bearing joint that is commonly injured. Osteoarthritis may develop after an injury, most commonly in women and especially in patients who are overweight. The knee is also an "emotional" joint. Most patients who have knee pain are deeply distressed not only by the pain but also by the resultant decrease in mobility and impact on their quality of life. Patients who were runners or athletes, or who enjoyed activities that require normal weight bearing find that they are unable to resume their normal or athletic activities. Patients who rely on activity to increase or maintain fitness and control their weight may also feel compromised.

The knee may be prone to unusual pain states, such as complex regional pain syndrome (CRPS). Many patients who undergo surgery experience damage to nerves, tissue, or blood vessels and develop severe pain syndromes that may defy interventional techniques to relieve the pain, including surgery, nerve blocks, epidural, sympathectomy (surgical removal of the sympathetic ganglion), or other procedures. The damage is often caused by the release of chemical substances that sensitize nerve endings during trauma, surgery, and/or stress. (Remember from early in the book that the release of noradrenaline and proinflammatory substances during the stress response can exacerbate pain. Researchers have found that the endocrine system stimulates a critical chemical pathway through which the human immune system is weakened by chronic stress.) Long-term damage may even occur from application of a tourniquet to reduce blood flow to the surgical site. The nerve most commonly affected by these scenarios is the infrapatella nerve.

Other symptoms that develop with CRPS are hypersensitivity, swelling, discoloration, thickening of joint surfaces, changes in skin and temperature, and loss of range of movement. Patients who have experienced a deep vein thrombosis after a surgical procedure may also be vulnerable to the condition.

CRPS somehow defies normal rehabilitation through the regular channels of physiotherapy, rehabilitation, and exercise regimens. However, it is now evident that many CRPS patients have benefited from treatment with acupuncture and electric currents. Furthermore, many clinical studies have been published that demonstrate resounding success in the treatment of osteoarthritis of the knee with acupuncture.

In 2001, at the meeting of the British Medical Acupuncture Society, Tukmachi et al. presented a report on a randomized, controlled trial of patients with osteoarthritis of the knee.[6] During the study, conducted at the Department of Rheumatology, Selly Oak Hospital, Birmingham University, patients were given electroacupuncture to the knee. Researchers concluded that acupuncture alleviates pain and reduces stiffness in osteoarthritis of the knee.

The points used were:

Acupuncture: Du 20, Li 4

Electroacupuncture: UB 40, UB 57, Xiyan, Sp 9, GB 34, St 36, Liv 3

In 2002, Broumas et al. conducted a study on patients older than sixty-five who were unable to receive anti-inflammatory medication due to gastrointestinal bleeding and renal deterioration.[7] The patients were treated with electroacupuncture combined with auricular (ear) acupuncture for knee pain. At 4 Hz the electroacupuncture treatment produced endorphins, and at 100 Hz it produced serotonin. The auricular acupuncture needle remained in the ear during the period of treatment. Seven sessions of acupuncture were given. It was found that the combination of electroacupuncture and auricular acupuncture was safe and effective in most patients. The results demonstrated an 80 percent improvement and resulted in satisfaction in the group of patients treated. Improvement lasted from one to seven months.

The acupoints used were: St 34 to 36, GB 33 to 34, Sp 10, Liv 7 to 8

Patients usually respond to a comprehensive approach when receiving acupuncture treatment for any condition in the knee. It is important to evaluate a patient's specific pain site. Most patients present with pain in various regions of the knee. A specific treatment should therefore be tailored for the individual. The sites that may present include one or more of the following:

◆ Patellofemoral joint

◆ Medial knee joint

◆ Infrapatella region

◆ Lateral joint line

◆ Quadriceps/hamstring/adductor/tensor fascia latae/iliotibial band/musculotendinous regions

◆ Posteromedial aspect of the knee joint

◆ Any injury site on the knee

The posterior aspect of the knee often presents with tenderness, weakness of the hamstring muscles, and joint stiffness. Treatment of the posteromedial aspect of the knee is crucial to most conditions where there is pain on the medial aspect of the knee, especially in osteoarthritis. Swelling is also a common feature of knee injury and disease.

The recommended points are:

Scalp: Du 20, leg region on the scalp motoric line (see diagram on page 174)

Ear points (see diagram on page 173): Shen Men (pain), sympathetic (if autonomic symptoms are present), knee region, point on the helix aligned with the knee, center point of the ear. It may be necessary to treat bilaterally to reach maximum improvement. It is helpful to insert and leave tiny indwelling needles in targeted points in the ear for continuing effects of treatment. These needles may be left in place for three to seven days. If irritation, pain, or infection occurs, the needles must be removed. The patient may be advised to press the needles gently three to five times a day and/or when pain occurs.

Distal points:

Si 3 on the opposite side of the body to the painful knee to improve mobility in the knee

Li 4 and Liv 3 bilaterally for improved mobility and relief of pain, depression, and anxiety

K3 bilaterally for knee pain, bone healing, and swelling

Local points:

A selection of the following: GB 34, St 32, 33, 34, 35, 36, Sp 9, 10, Liv 8, point Heding (superior to the patella), UB 36, 38, 40, 57

Needle penetration from outer Xiyan (St 35) to inner Xiyan point: A long needle may be inserted to reach the medial side from under the lateral aspect of the patella tendon. Care must be taken to avoid penetration of the skin on the medial side. This treatment eases pain under and inferior to the patella.

Needles surrounding the patella: eight needles placed superficially at an angle be-

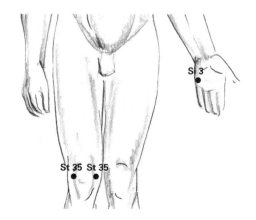

tween fifteen and thirty degrees to the skin. This technique relieves inflammation, induration, and pain underneath and around the patella.

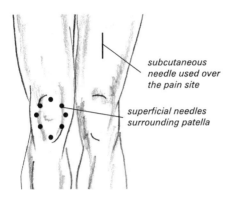

subcutaneous needle used over the pain site

superficial needles surrounding patella

Needles inserted subcutaneously into painful regions: These needles may have an effect on the A-beta and A-delta receptors in the afferent nerves and may block pain signals to the spinal cord and brain. The patient is encouraged to perform active movements after this application. The needles may be left taped in position for seventy-two hours.

Plum-blossom needling may relieve swelling and reduce thickening of the tissues, especially after surgical procedures when hematomas or thickening has accumulated.

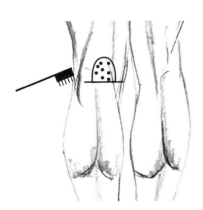

Periosteal pecking will relieve unusual pain, especially at a bony point. Care must be taken not to traumatize bone or underlying tissue.

Needles surrounding a relatively small area of swelling, induration, or pain may be inserted at a thirty-degree angle around the area. Another needle is then inserted perpendicularly into the center of the area.

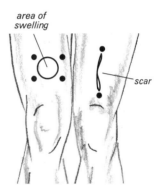

area of swelling

scar

Scar: Acupuncture can be applied at the arthroscopy site, on any surgical scar, or at the point of injury.

Electroacupuncture may be used appropriately on the above points or regions.

D. Headaches

Headaches are a common complaint and may be of circulatory or neurological origin. Certain conditions are associated with headaches, such as cluster and migraine headaches, trigeminal neuralgia, and tension. These headaches are benign in that no brain tumors or infection is present.

Acupuncture is mostly used to treat the areas of muscle spasm and the regions of referral that are present in most tension-type headaches. Muscle spasm that creates nerve compression in the intervertebral foramen may affect the occipital nerve supplying the muscles in the head. This may produce headaches or trigger points in these muscles. Headaches are often accompanied by cervical (neck) stiffness in these conditions.

The common points for headache are:

Du 20   for relaxation

Du 14   improves cervical extension

EP 1   for relaxation and central forehead pain

GB 20   alleviates any pain in the head

GB 21   releases trapezius muscle spasm

Bai lao   releases muscle spasm, stiffness, pain, and headache

Any other tender areas that may affect headaches may also be included.

Distal points that influence headaches:

Li 4   relieves headaches that may result from constipation or emanate from the facial region, especially the lower jaw, and relieves pain in any area of the body

Lu 7   relieves pain emanating from the lung meridian

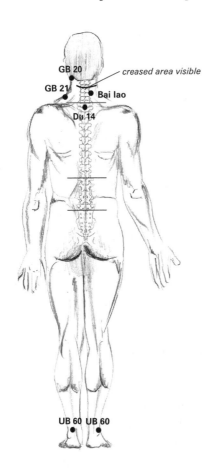

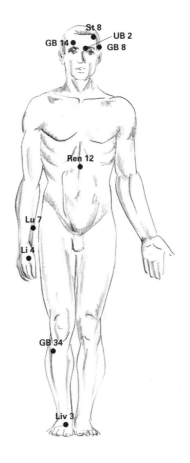

Sp 6	relaxes muscles and relieves stress
GB 34	relaxes ligaments, tendons, and muscles
Liv 3	relieves depression and pain
UB 60	relieves pain in the urinary bladder meridian that passes centrally over the head and neck
Ren 12	relieves abdominal disorders that affect headaches
St 8	especially for pain relief in the temporalis muscle
St 36 and St44	relieves stomach disorders that may precipitate headaches
St 44	relieves dream-disturbed sleep as a result of heavy meals

Many patients have poor posture, or have sedentary occupations that cause them to adopt poor head posture (forward head posture). Poor posture compromises joint structures and diminishes the natural anterior curve of the neck. This produces a straight cervical spine (stressing C5/6/7) with an increase in extension of the uppermost vertebrae C2/3. This creates spasm and shortening in the muscles of the neck and thoracic spine. If this position is maintained over a period of years, creases may develop in the back of the neck, which may indicate the area of maximal compression on the cervical joints. There is often an increase in the thoracic kyphosis to compensate for the forward head posture (dowager's hump).

Acupuncture may be applied into these creases if the patient has headaches and one or more creases in the neck region. Deep needling into the crease, either bilaterally at C5/6 near the spinous process, or slightly laterally in line with these transverse processes (this point may be on or close to Bai lao), produces relief from headaches caused by bony changes present in such patients. These creases may also be present at C2, and this area may be needled in the same manner.

Local points between the vertebrae, which cause pain and stiffness, will also relieve pain. Many cervical headaches relate to tenderness in the trapezius (mostly upper trapezius) muscle. Needling these tender points relieves the condition.

Needling into the following areas of referral also reduces pain:

◆ Local needling into the occipital muscles situated posteriorly (at the back of the skull), with low- or high-frequency electroacupuncture of 4 or 200 Hz, respectively, relaxes these muscles

◆ GB 20, 21—classical points for head pain and headache

◆ UB 2, EP 1, GB 14—in the forehead, for pain in the frontalis muscles

◆ SJ 23, GB 1—area surrounding the eyes for temporal or parietal pain

◆ St 5, 6, 7; SJ 21, 23; GB 2, 3—for the jaw region for temporomandibular joint problems

◆ GB 8, St 8 for the temporalis region

◆ St 9, 10; Si 17; Li 17, 18—assist when pain occurs in the sternocleidomastoid muscles (cervical whiplash)

IMS can also be applied to any of these muscles to relax spasm.

E. Neuralgia

"Neuralgia" is the term used to describe pain in a nerve that has been attacked by a virus, as in postherpetic neuralgia (shingles). Trigeminal neuralgia is caused by a virus or inflammation attacking the trigeminal nerve; brachial neuralgia is caused by a virus attacking a branch of the brachial plexus, with ensuing pain and weakness. Neuralgias may also be brought about by disease processes, such as diabetes, where nerve endings are destroyed or damaged, and pain, uncomfortable sensations, and weakness develop.

Acupuncture can assist with many neuralgic conditions, if the area of the affected nerve (possibly spinal) and the area of referral are treated.

In postherpetic neuralgia of a thoracic nerve, the patient may present with burning, sharp, shooting pain in the region of the rib cage (often thoracic—T8 to T10). Needles may be inserted into the central spinal region (T8 and/or T10) and into the area of referral. Electroacupuncture with low frequency (4 Hz) and/or followed by high frequency (100–200 Hz) relieves the pain. Electric currents (discussed in Chapter 8) may also be applied to this painful region.

F. Wound/Scar Pain

Many wounds or postsurgical scars become painful. The pain may present in the form of sensitivity to touch and may spread in a global fashion under the scar and into the surrounding tissue. This pain may refer distally, produce unusual pain states, and also become shooting, burning, and/or electrical. Such pain may be due to the formation of a neuroma (benign), as previously mentioned, in the area where there has been a surgical incision and/or underlying soft tissue, or muscle. The ancient Chinese belief was that a scar or injury could develop "toxicity" within the wound, which was not an indication of infection but rather was related to irritation and/or inflammation.

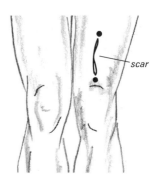

Needles may be inserted in either end of the scar or in areas in the scar that are identified as specifically tender. Electroacupuncture at low frequency (2–4 Hz) may be used and may then be followed by higher frequencies (100–200 Hz), if pain persists.

A scar often indicates that the underlying tissue is unhealthy, especially when the scar is red, thickened, or closing unevenly. Acupuncture heals the scar and improves the health of the underlying tissue. Successful treatment will cause the scar to fade and heal with no adhesion forming in the underlying tissue. Moreover, the surrounding and underlying ligaments, tendons, muscles, and joints will also become mobile and relieved of pain. Pain that may have referred from the scar to unusual areas, often far removed from the scar, may also dissipate with this treatment.

G. Sympathetically Mediated Pain

Sympathetically mediated pain originates from the sympathetic nervous system and manifests as spontaneous pain following nerve injury. There is functional evidence of a direct link between sympathetic terminals that release noradrenaline and the sensory neurons. A recommended protocol for sympathetically mediated pain successfully used by Linda Rapson and others follows:[8]

Auricular (ear) points usually treated bilaterally:

◆ Shen Men (parasympathetic)

◆ Autonomic point—sympathetic

◆ Region of pain represented in the ear—usually the toe, foot, ankle, knee, leg, finger, hand, wrist, arm, elbow, or specific spinal region

◆ Point on the helix of the ear at the level of the painful body region

◆ Center point of the ear

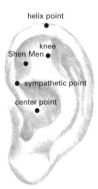

helix point

knee
Shen Men

sympathetic point

center point

Movement is encouraged in the painful peripheral region immediately after these points have been needled. Many patients report a sensation in the affected limb or area during the needling.

The following sympathetic switches that may be relevant to the area of disuse or injury should also be selected:

SNS	PNS
St 36	H 7
Li 4	Sp 6
Liv 3	UB 23
GB 20	UB 10
Du 26	Sacral points applicable to the region: UB 31–34
Du14	

If necessary, another regimen (in the scalp) that has produced effective results may be followed in addition to or instead of the aforementioned points:

Scalp points, bilateral where appropriate:

◆ Du 20

◆ Shishencong

◆ EP 1

Motoric or sensory line representing the area of the pain

Many of these points produce relaxation and expression of emotion (tears, outbursts of emotion, and increased communication). Movement of the affected part is encouraged during this needle insertion.

Local areas may be targeted with electroacupuncture treatment around the affected area. In a joint, such as the knee, four points are used—two needles superior and two needles inferior to the knee—in nonspecific and nonpainful areas. This permits the current to pass through the affected region, usually produces relief from pain and sensitivity, and improves movement.

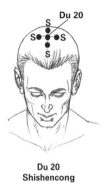

Du 20
Shishencong

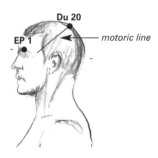

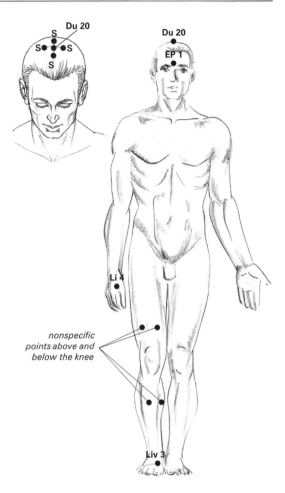

Similarly, nonspecific, nonpainful points can be used superiorly and inferiorly on the meridians that pass over the nerve supply to the knee joint.

Sympathetically mediated pain (SMP) may become unstable or unreliable in its response to treatment. At some stage in its development, but not always, this type of pain may be mediated by the sympathetic nervous system. Changes in the sympathetic nervous system (SNS) may occur due to ongoing pain. If the system becomes nonresponsive to treatment of the SNS, changes in the nervous system occur, producing sympathetically independent pain (SIP). When this happens, there is a complex mix of symptoms, in which the local region of injury (possibly the central/spinal nerve, as in patients with spinal cord injuries, or peripheral/wrist, as in a Colles fracture) and its nerve

pathway become hypersensitive. An aberration in the nerve conduction occurs, and abnormal messages are sent to the local and central nerve supply (peripheral, spinal, and brain). The result is a combination of symptoms of severe and unusual pain, swelling, discoloration, temperature changes, and, possibly, skin hypersensitivity (cannot touch the skin due to severe pain). Changes take place from skin to bone, and psychological changes, such as depression and anxiety, may even manifest.

In effect, patients with these types of conditions are best treated with a combination of therapies, discussed in detail in the chapter on multimodal treatment.

H. Deafferentation, or "Burning" Pain

Deafferentation, or *"burning" pain,* refers to pain that is deafferented, that is, where control by the central nervous system has diminished, due to either partial or complete severance or damage to the nerve, as in spinal cord injuries. This type of pain can also occur as a result of injuries or diseases that don't involve the spinal cord; for example:

◆ Trauma

◆ Postsurgery

◆ Postherpetic neuralgia

◆ Trigeminal neuralgia

◆ Burning tongue syndrome

◆ Multiple sclerosis

◆ Guillain-Barré syndrome

◆ Transverse myelitis

◆ Cervical myelopathy

◆ Syringomyelia

◆ Chronic inflammatory demyelinating polyneuropathy

◆ Arteriovenous malformation

◆ Arachnoiditis

◆ Paraneoplastic encephalomyelitis

The following treatment regimen may be used for all types of "burning" pain:

Du 18

Du 20

Du 21

EP 1

The needles are inserted at a shallow angle along the meridian, from posterior to anterior. Electrostimulation is given at 1 Hz for thirty minutes, five times per week, with treatment decreasing as the effects accumulate. Electrical connections are made to Du 18 and 20, Du 21, and EP 1.

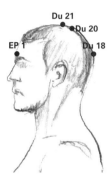

Patients who respond poorly to this regimen may improve once a course of amytriptyline (an antidepressant) is introduced. Amytriptyline is synergistic (helps or promotes improvement) with acupuncture.

The pain is usually of a burning nature but may also include sensations that are lancinating (feeling like a lance has been pushed into the skin), sharp, paroxysmal (sudden but usually not long-lasting), or stabbing in nature. Such pain may respond poorly to the usual pain medications. Antidepressants and anticonvulsants have, however, been effective in cases of burning, shooting, paroxysmal pain. This type of pain demonstrates changes in the central nervous system affecting the brain and spinal cord.

Sharp, paroxysmal pain is similar to that emanating from a neuroma (benign growth on the nerve), where the reaction from the nerve is similar to that occurring in an "epileptic fit."

The Jingwell points are often included in the treatment of severe pain as described above, especially burning pain on the tendinomuscular meridians (energy lines passing over the muscles and tendons). These points are behind the corner of the toenail or fingernail, either medially or laterally, depending on the meridian involved. These points are painful to stimulate, yet have profound effects on the psyche and physical body. After insertion of a needle into this point, pain and unusual sensations may diminish within thirty seconds. The needles may be left in situ for a relatively short period of about two to three minutes.

Any other acupuncture points that may assist in relieving the pain are also included in the treatment protocol. A multimodal approach is highly successful with most patients.

I. Tendinomuscular Meridian Pain

This section deals with tendinomuscular meridian pain in spinal cord and peripheral nerve injury.

In 1999, L. M. Rapson conducted a retrospective study of three hundred patients who had experienced pain for anywhere from two weeks to fifteen years and who were treated by electroacupuncture.[9] The best response was reported in patients with constant, bilateral, burning pain. These patients were treated by inserting needles on the midline of the scalp, accompanied by low frequency (1 Hz) electrical stimulation.

In another study of thirty-five patients receiving tendinomuscular acupuncture on the Jingwell points, seventeen reported a VAS score of 100 percent relief, others experienced 75–90 percent relief, some experienced 50–70 percent relief, and a small number had an improvement of less than 45 percent.[10]

A CASE HISTORY FROM RESEARCHER L.M. RAPSON OF A FORTY-YEAR-OLD MALE PATIENT

The patient was an incomplete quadriplegic at cervical 7 (C7), who became a complete quadriplegic after an atrioventricular bleed. Three subsequent surgeries produced some recovery of function, but severe burning pain developed in the left arm. This pain was present for four years but was aggravated by the use of other therapies. Even conventional acupuncture approaches failed.

The patient complained of pain in the left hand, third finger, wrist, forearm, elbow, triceps, axilla, and scapula. The pain pattern was represented by the tendinomuscular meridians of the small intestine, triple warmer, large intestine, pericardium, and lung.

Treatment

◆ Jingwell points for two to three minutes

Total effect of the first treatment

◆ Increased warmth in the arm, feet, and the rest of the body, with the patient reporting, "It feels like heaven!"

◆ Lightening of a dark patch on the skin of the forearm

◆ Increased range of movement in the wrist and fingers

◆ Disappearance of spasms of the wrist

◆ "Cardboard" feeling (the sensation experienced by a patient that the body is made of stiff cardboard with no feeling in it) lowered from clavicle to nipples

◆ Pain relief lasting eight hours

◆ Increased energy and concentration

This treatment regimen continued and other points on the relevant meridians were also included.

As a result, the patient experienced improved sleep and pain relief that persisted for two or three days. Many memories surfaced during the treatment, the "cardboard" feeling disappeared from the chest, improved wrist movement remained, and the patient could consistently remove pain with self-treatment on Jingwell points, using a TENS pointer. The patient still has pain in damp weather and experiences a foggy feeling in the head, as well as spells of confusion.

J. Integrative Neuromuscular Acupoint System

A discussion of acupuncture for pain management would be incomplete without mention of an innovative and effective design named the integrative neuromuscular acupoint system (INMAS).[11] This approach incorporates the principles of both Eastern and Western acupuncture. Its value lies in the fact that it allows treatment of the whole person—body plus spirit/psyche—without having to have full knowledge of traditional Chinese medicine, yet with enough information to use points that affect the whole body, for example, for nausea (Pericardium 6) or for the immune system (Du 14, Li 11, Sp 36, St 6).

The results can easily be replicated as the same protocol can be applied to most patients (nonspecificity). INMAS combines the use of homeostatic acupoints for the immune system, symptomatic acupoints in the region of the pain, and paravertebral acupoints for the nerve supply, either to the somatosensory or the sympathetic nerves supplying the affected region. This combi-

nation is an accurate and fully encompassing therapy that treats the area of the problem (e.g., lower back), the nerve supply to the region affected, and homeostatic points that balance the immune, autonomic, metabolic, and emotional disturbances either precipitated by or influencing the condition or region.

6. Periosteal Pecking for Burning Pain and Inflammation

Periosteal (bone) pecking involves delicately tapping the bone with an acupuncture needle. The treatment benefits inflamed joints, bone surfaces, and intransigent and often burning pain, especially on the spinal joints. It stimulates the descending pain-control mechanisms and elicits endorphins and anti-inflammatories. It may produce a profound histamine reaction (released in response to an injury with an antibody-antigen reaction) with unusual but accurate pain referrals. It also improves mobility.

Many patients experience a type of burning pain that is different from that described by patients with centralized disturbance. This type of burning pain occurs typically in inflammatory conditions, especially in a joint or bone. Whether the joint is spinal or peripheral (knee, wrist), patients commonly describe pain across the mid-back region, especially after standing or performing physical activities such as cooking/baking. The thoracic spine may have been flexed for prolonged periods, creating muscle spasm in the affected region.

The interesting thing about this pain is that it often refers to unusual areas; for example:

- proximal to (above) a specific region, e.g., thoracic 4 or 5, into the cervical (neck) muscles, or head, as in a headache or a strange sensation in the head

- ache in the arms, often generalized, or as tingling or numbness

- opposite side of the afflicted area of the thoracic spine

- superior or inferior to the region affected

- pain, tingling, or numbness in the legs

The therapist often fails to appreciate the significance of these referring pains or sensations described by the patient, until after this type of needle insertion has elicited the sensation previously experienced and mentioned by the patient.

Anatomical textbooks provide no explicit charts of this type of unusual referral. One explanation is that such referred pain may arise from inflammatory chemicals sensitizing nerve endings in the local or spinal cord area (to which it is closely situated). The sympathetic nervous system (SNS) may also become involved in this pain, as the SNS may refer to as many as six levels above or below the pain or injury site. The outer layer of the bone—the periosteum—is richly supplied with blood vessels and nerves, any one of which can create pain and, more importantly, be manipulated to *relieve* the pain.

Periosteal pecking is usually performed on a bone that is prominent and superficial. The most sensitive area of bone in the spine is often the spinous process or transverse process. This area is tapped for thirty seconds or less, with great care taken not to traumatize blood vessels or nerve endings with the acupuncture needle.

7. Plum-Blossom Needling for Indurated Swelling and Pain

The ancient Chinese technique of plum-blossom needling releases interstitial fluid, which eases stiffness and/or localized, indurated swelling and sensitivity in a joint or region. It also improves mobility. A counter-irritation—pain—is produced that stimulates descending mechanisms from the brain to block the pain in the spinal cord. The plum-blossom needle resembles a hammer with seven tiny needles embedded in the upper portion. The needles are briefly tapped on the skin over the painful or swollen site (see page 169), until the skin appears to break down and tiny drops of blood are released. A suction cup is placed over the area, drawing blood and tissue fluid from the underlying tissue, which collects in the cup. This technique requires a sterile approach.

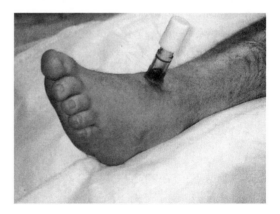

According to traditional Chinese textbooks, this application was used for treatment of the nervous system, headaches, dizziness, vertigo, insomnia, the skin, gastrointestinal diseases, gynecological diseases, painful joints, and paralysis.

"Cupping" has long been used in Europe for many ailments. It entails the use of glass or plastic cups that are attached to the skin through an applied negative pressure via a suction handle or a flame inserted into the cup, creating a vacuum. When applied over an area that has been tapped by the plum-blossom, the cupping creates local congestion, which causes exudates to be released through the skin from the interstitial tissue. The fluid that is released does not emanate from a deep joint or structure, but rather from the local soft tissue that may have been traumatized or injured and has developed into a thickened hematoma. Often, releasing a few drops of fluid or blood relieves pressure in this area and results in pain relief and improved mobility. It has been postulated that the pain relief may result from the following mechanisms:

- Counter-irritation produced from the painful pricking of the skin, which may stimulate the descending pain-control mechanisms emanating from the brain centers
- Release of pressure and fluid in the interstitial tissue[12]

8. Subcutaneous Needling Over Painful Areas

This type of needling involves the superficial placement of a needle under the skin. The length of the needle that penetrates the skin must be felt under the whole area. Initially, the needle is uncomfortable to insert, because it passes through the nerve fibers in the skin that relay pain messages to the spinal cord and brain. Once the needle has been inserted, however, the initial pain subsides and the treatment produces pain relief over the painful or sensitive region and permits improved range of motion within the tissue itself, including the underlying joints. The pain relief may be due to stimulation of the pain-blocking and counter-irritant pathways. This technique should *not* be used on areas that are hypersensitive to touch.

Subcutaneous needling may have an effect similar to that achieved by transcutaneous electrical nerve stimulation (TENS), except that there is no movement or stimulation of the needle. It is similar to placing a hand over the painful site, but in this case the "hand" is in the skin itself!

A carefully selected area must be chosen for this treatment, in order to avoid traumatizing or damaging the skin or underlying tissue.

9. Intramuscular Stimulation (IMS) Needling for Muscle Spasm

Intramuscular needling, as advocated by C. Chan Gunn, involves a deep and direct needle insertion.[13] It is indicated by examination of the radicular (nerve) or segmental pattern of the problem, which could be related to pressure on a nerve, as in spondylosis, leading to pain in a musculoskeletal region. The problem could also be related to referral into a primary or secondary trigger point or into a limb.

According to Gunn, muscle shortening, autonomic changes, and pain are natural occurrences in radiculopathy (compressed nerve). Shortened or tight muscles cause narrowing of intervertebral foramina, creating indirect irritation of the nerve root.

Myofascial pain refers to tender areas that exist primarily in the muscles. Needle insertion into the motor points of the tender areas produces a muscle twitch that will relieve pain in radiculopathy and many other musculoskeletal and neuropathic pain conditions. As there are many layers of muscles, pain relief may occur when each of these layers containing areas of tenderness is deeply needled.

Once the twitch response has been elicited, the needle may be withdrawn, or it may be left in place for ten to twenty minutes, especially if it remains grasped by the muscle twitch for some minutes. Electrical stimulation (via TENS) may also be applied to needles used in painful and tight musculoskeletal areas. Many patients with severe muscle spasm, especially in the paraspinal musculature, find great relief from this technique.

◆ ◆ ◆

The most effective physical treatments are combinations of electrotherapy and acupuncture. Massage and mobilization are also very important aspects of any treatment regimen, but acupuncture and electrotherapy are fast acting, often producing instant and lasting pain relief and improved mobility. The value of acupuncture in improving mobility is evident as an immediate and visible change in movement and pain perception. This is rarely observed with other modalities.

Most conditions are relieved by using the same acupoints, as acupuncture treats the symptoms of many different diseases with the same acupoints. Pain does not always occur in simple or accessible areas; it may become complex and referred, or it may change its nature and quality. It is therefore impossible to describe protocols for every painful condition or every treatment regimen. The guidelines mentioned above, however, will target the problem at any stage of its manifestation.

TREATMENT WITH TENS

A TENS device may be used in the clinic by the therapist on the patient. The patient may also use the device independently, outside the clinic, usually on the advice of the therapist. Once the therapist decides that the patient would benefit from home use of TENS, the therapist must advise the patient on the correct position of the electrodes and also provide different options that may enhance pain relief. When the pain changes, the therapist must advise the patient on the best positioning of the electrodes as progress is made.

A TENS unit is a low-voltage, battery-operated electrical device. It has a biphasic alternating current with a zero net direct-current component that does not produce a buildup of ions of negative or positive polarity under either electrode.

It is compact and can be clipped to a belt or placed in a pocket. It usually has dual channels with two leads attached to each channel. Each lead has both a positive and a negative wire, indicated by a red or black marker. Electrodes are attached to each wire on the lead. The best electrodes are adhesive and make close contact with the skin. Most TENS units are equipped with their own rubber electrodes with adhesive attachments; these usually do not remain sticky for very long. It is recommended that the user obtain extra electrodes that are more adhesive or change the electrodes frequently to maintain good contact with the skin.

Adherence to personal preferences is important for the comfort of the patient and relief of the condition. A patient should have the opportunity to try different frequencies (1–200 Hz), widths (50–250 milliseconds), and pulse modes (constant, burst, or modulation). Over many years of TENS use, I have observed that most patients prefer the protocols described below. Patients may, however, change the parameters if comfort and pain relief are not achieved after following these recommendations.

Patients who find that rubbing eases their pain may be "good contenders" for TENS use. These patients may already have programmed their systems by rubbing and otherwise stimulating the A-beta fibers—that is, achieving relief by eliciting their own pain-relieving neurotransmitters.

Important Information about the Use of TENS

♦ High-frequency TENS stimulates the release of dynorphin, enkephalin, and serotonin in the spinal region and brain.

♦ Low-frequency TENS stimulates the release of endorphins in various areas of the nervous system.

♦ The effects of TENS are cumulative in certain TENS responders. Long-term use of TENS may produce over 60 percent improvement in the condition. Other people, however, find that the effectiveness of TENS diminishes over time.

♦ When TENS is successful in relieving a patient's pain in one area of the body, it will usually have positive effects in other areas.

♦ TENS can be used for both *acute* and *chronic* pain.

♦ TENS used immediately after the pain occurs will be more effective in a shorter period of time.

♦ Ideally, TENS should be used for eight hours a day for three consecutive days, to determine whether the patient is a "complete TENS responder."

♦ Recommended dosage: To achieve the most comfort on a painful site, TENS should be used on modulation mode at a frequency of 200 Hz (highest frequency possible on the device) with a width of 80 milliseconds.

♦ TENS current sensation is usually experienced between 3 and 4 milliamps in normal tissue.

♦ TENS should be used for a minimum period of forty minutes to produce effective changes in the pain.

♦ Patients should use TENS routinely during their daily work, sport, or recreation activities.

♦ TENS can relieve pain from the sympathetic nervous system, producing improvement in circulation and movement.

♦ If TENS increases pain, *stop* using it. It could make the condition worse.

Recommendations for the Use of TENS

♦ One or two channels should be used, depending on the area of the pain.

♦ The negative electrode (attached to the black connection) is applied to the pain site.

♦ The positive electrode (attached to the red connection) may be placed above, below, or to the side of the pain site.

♦ The electrodes of opposite polarity may be placed in close proximity to each other, or at any convenient distance apart, but should *not* come into contact with each other.

♦ Electrodes that adhere properly and comfortably to the body should be used.

♦ To avoid interruption of sleep and movement of the electrodes that may produce unexpected, uncomfortable sensations, patients should not sleep with TENS.

♦ The TENS current should be strong enough to interfere with the pain sensation, but not so strong that it produces discomfort.

♦ If muscular contractions occur, there should be no discomfort or uncontrollable muscular twitching.

♦ Tissues adapt to electric currents. If the current appears to decrease, increase it once again to a comfort level.

♦ If the current has to be increased to a maximum of 10 milliamps, change the battery.

◆ Pain will diminish in area and intensity as relief occurs.

◆ If the pain changes, follow the pain. If it moves from a lateral or outer region to the center of the spine, for example, move the electrodes to the new pain site. Continue to follow the pain until it disappears.

◆ Use TENS along anatomical nerve pathways, following the nerve supply to the painful region to achieve best results.

◆ If a region is extremely sensitive to touch, it may be too painful to place the TENS over it. Place the electrodes above and below the site until sensitivity diminishes.

◆ If a patient presents with any or all of the following sympathetic symptoms: severe pain, sweating, temperature changes, discoloration, swelling, and/or stiffness, place TENS electrodes on the sympathetic supply to the affected region on the spine, or from the sympathetic nerve supply to above the painful region, or on the somatic nerve supply on the spine to above the painful region.

◆ If a large area of the spine is painful, use long rubber electrodes (see diagrams on page 188), either in the center of the spine or on either side of the painful region.

◆ TENS may be combined simultaneously with other treatment modalities, including other electrical treatments (e.g., hot/ice pack, sequential faradic current/NMES, modified direct current, and acupuncture, with or without electrical stimulation).

◆ TENS may create pain over a recent fracture site, due to vibration of unstable bone fragments, but once all movement of the bone is no longer possible, TENS may be safely and comfortably used.

◆ When used on acupuncture needles, TENS is executed at a low frequency of 1–4 Hz, at a width of up to 250 milliseconds, and in the burst mode. It can also be used as an acupuncture-type treatment without needles, using only electrodes.

◆ Treatment with acupuncture needles may commence with a low frequency for twenty minutes, followed by a high frequency for a further twenty minutes, to elicit all the different natural pain relievers present in the system.

◆ See modified direct current (Appendix C) for alternative TENS placements in certain treatments.

Rules of TENS

◆ The electrodes of opposite polarities may be placed close together but not in contact with one another. If they touch, the current will not pass through the body but rather through the electrodes.

◆ The electrodes may be placed anywhere on the external surface of the body, except on the areas mentioned in Chapter 8 as contraindicated or as ineffective.

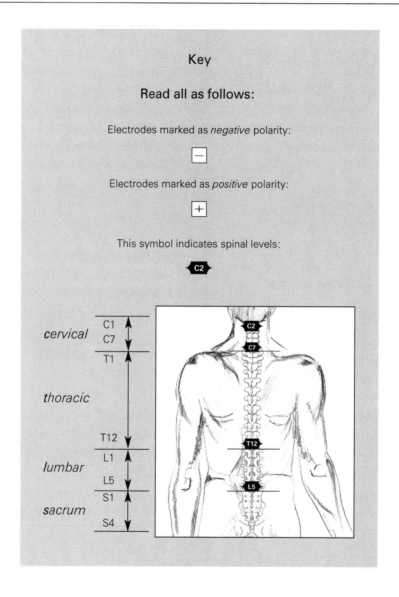

Key

Read all as follows:

Electrodes marked as *negative* polarity:

$-$

Electrodes marked as *positive* polarity:

$+$

This symbol indicates spinal levels:

C2

cervical — C1, C7
T1

thoracic

T12
L1
lumbar — L5
S1
sacrum — S4

All treatments may be used for a protracted period (eight hours daily for three days, or for at least forty minutes per day), if convenient. Any configuration of placement may be used that will block the pain either locally or centrally on any pain site (except, again, those sites that are contraindicated). Many other placements or suggestions for treatment may be adapted from the instructions for placement of electrodes in modified direct current (see Appendix C). TENS may also be used internally to reduce anal or vaginal pain (mostly neuropathic). Specific electrodes are used for these applications. The scope of this topic is not addressed in this book.

TENS Electrode-Placement Diagrams

1. TENS Electrode Placement: Treatment of the Pain Site

Place the negative electrode on the pain site and the positive electrode adjacent to it or on a nerve supply to the painful region.

For example:

Lumbar spine at L4/5 with 4 electrodes

or

the hamstring muscle in the leg with 2 electrodes

or

the deltoid muscle of the shoulder with 2 electrodes

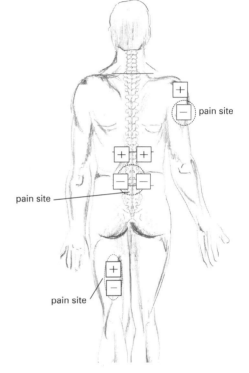

2. TENS Electrode Placement: If the Pain Site Is Hypersensitive

TENS may irritate the condition if applied directly on the pain site; in that case, apply TENS indirectly.

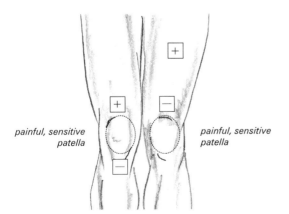

For example:

Pain site—patella on the knee joint with electrodes placed as follows:

Positive electrode above and negative electrode below the patella

or

Both positive and negative electrodes placed only above the patella

3. TENS Electrode Placement: If the Pain Site Is Hypersensitive

TENS may irritate the condition if applied directly on the pain site; in that case, apply TENS on the spinal nerve supply to the painful area.

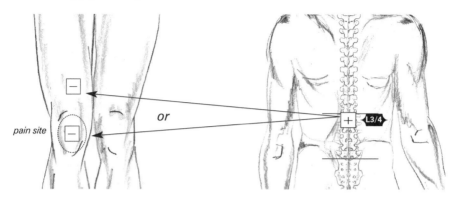

For example:

Positive electrode placed at L3/4 (spinal nerve supply to the knee), and negative electrode placed either on or above the patella; 2 or 4 electrodes may be used in this placement

4. TENS Electrode Placement: If the Pain Site Is Hypersensitive and If Sympathetic Symptoms Are Present

TENS may irritate the condition if applied directly on the pain site; therefore, apply TENS on the sympathetic nervous system and above or below the affected area (e.g., knee).

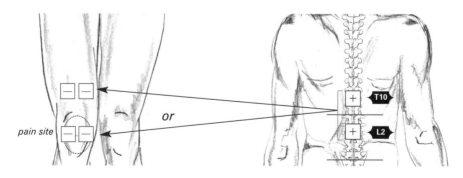

For example:

Positive electrodes (2) placed on T10 and L2 (sympathetic nerve supply to the low back and legs) and negative electrodes (2) placed either on or above the patella

5. TENS Electrode Placement: If the Pain Site Is Hypersensitive and Sensitization Has Occurred

TENS may irritate the condition if applied directly on or near the pain site; therefore, for knee pain, apply TENS *only* to the spinal nerve supply and to the SNS supply to the low back and leg.

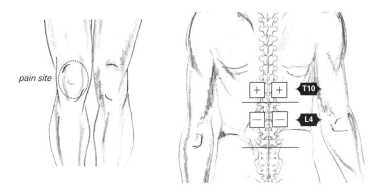

For example:

Positive electrodes (2) placed superiorly at T10 and negative electrodes (2) placed inferiorly on L3/4, depending on the level of the somatic and SNS supply to the specific pain site

If any symptoms of disturbance of the sympathetic nervous system are present—such as unusual or severe pain, sweating, temperature changes, swelling, discoloration, and/or stiffness anywhere in the body—treat the SNS with the placement of electrodes in the region of the SNS that supplies the pain site.

T1–5   supplies head, neck, and arms

T1–10   supplies thoracic region

T10–L2 supplies low back and legs

6. TENS Electrode Placement: The Treatment of Pain in Large Areas of the Spine Using Large (Rubber or Other Type) Electrodes

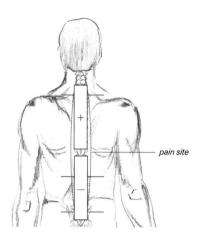

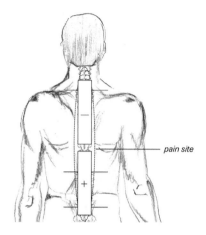

For treatment of pain along the whole spinal area, use 2 electrodes

◆ positive electrode superior and negative electrode inferior

or

for most pain in the lower region of the spine, use 2 electrodes

◆ positive electrode superior and negative electrode inferior

For treatment of pain along the whole spinal area with most pain in the upper region of the spine, use 2 electrodes

◆ positive electrode inferior and negative electrode superior

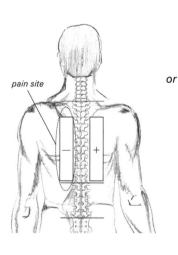

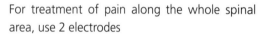

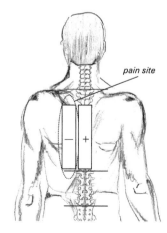

For treatment of pain along a large spinal area with most pain originating on the left side of the spinal area

◆ negative electrode placed on the relevant areas of most pain, and positive electrode placed

– at the same levels on the right-hand side of the spine

or

– on the center of the spine

Specific Treatments Using TENS

Pain Centrally or Unilaterally at L5

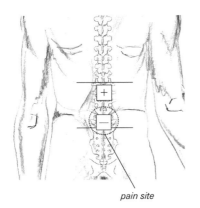

pain site

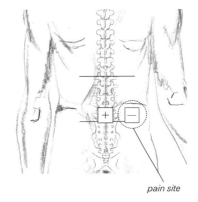

pain site

*Treatment of pain at L5 **centrally***

◆ placing the positive electrode superiorly at L3/4 and the negative inferiorly at L5/S1
or

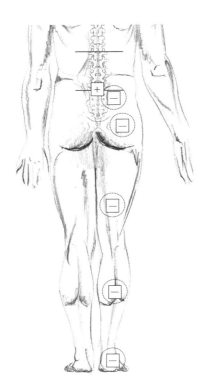

unilaterally

◆ placing the positive electrode at L4/5 centrally and the negative electrode adjacent on the painful side (right L4/5 facet joint region)

Pain Referred from L5/S1 into Sacroiliac Joint, Buttocks, Leg, and/or Feet

Place the positive electrode centrally at L5/S1 and the negative electrode on the area of referred pain (right sacroiliac joint, gluteus muscle, thigh, calf, or foot).

Treat the specific area (right or left) of pain, and follow the pain as it recedes toward the center, in the spine.

The same principles are applied to other regions of the spine.

Pain in the Jaw after Teeth Surgery

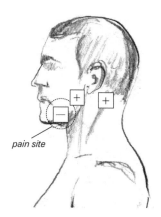

Place the negative electrode on the pain site on the jaw and the positive electrode adjacent to it or on the nerve (facial nerve) or nerve root (C2) supplying the facial muscles.

Pain after Healed Fracture of the Clavicle

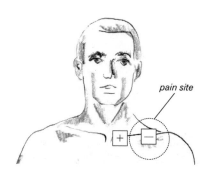

Place the negative electrode on the most painful site and the positive electrode adjacent to it, in a convenient position.

Pain Referred from Thoracic Spine or Costovertebral Joints into the Anterior Chest Wall

Place the positive electrodes on the right thoracic (costovertebral) region (T4–8)

or

centrally at this level and the negative electrodes anteriorly on the chest wall in the region of the painful ribs.

or

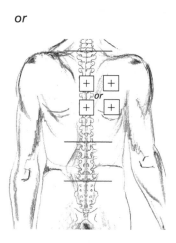

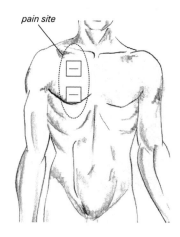

For Pain in Both the Costovertebral Region and the Anterior Chest Wall

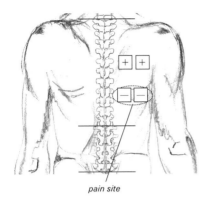
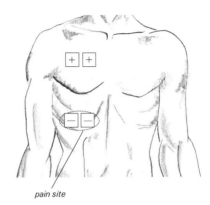

pain site   *pain site*

Place the positive electrode (1–2) superior to the pain and the negative electrode (1–2) locally on the pain sites—posteriorly on the thoracic region and anteriorly on the chest wall.

Combining TENS and Modified Direct Current (MDC) Treatment

Pain in the Medial Aspect of the Knee

■ = TENS   ▲ = MDC

For example:

Place the positive TENS electrode centrally on the patella and the negative electrode on the medial pain site of the knee joint. At the same time, place the 2 negative electrodes of the MDC on the medial side and the 2 positive electrodes of the MDC on the lateral side of the knee joint.

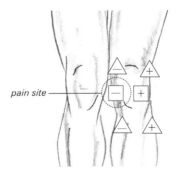

pain site

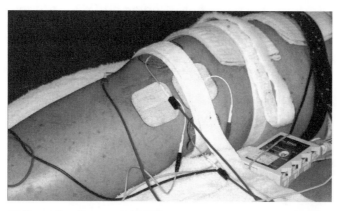

TENS and Faradic current (NMES)

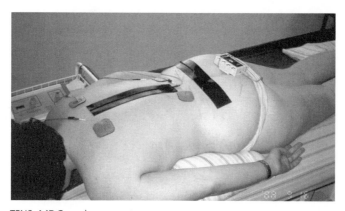

TENS, MDC, and acupuncture

In 1974, Norman Shealy, a neurosurgeon and protagonist of TENS, commented as follows in the medical journal *Emergency Medicine:*

Taken all in all, TENS is completely safe and it can be used universally, subject to instruction and the caution that it should not be used in cases of persistent pain without medical advice. Most certainly it should be standard in every emergency room facility. My feeling is that it should be used in every single pain state and it should be the first treatment of acute pain, even before drugs.[1]

Although the quote is over thirty years old, it contains very wise words because in the ensuing years this insight has been lost. Only now are people beginning to use TENS effectively. Many more patients need to have information about TENS treatment so they, too, can reach for this "electrical pill" as a first line of defense against pain.

TREATMENT WITH MDC

Treatment Effects on Different Regions of the Body

GENERAL TREATMENT (Rx)	LOCAL TREATMENT
1. 6 Rx on the spine (any selected levels)	**1. 1–12 Rx**
Effects:	*Effects:*
– Pain relief – Improved mobility – Improved circulation – Decreased anxiety – Possible immune enhancement – Other effects	– Pain relief – Improved mobility – Decreased swelling – Reduced muscle spasm – Reduced paresthesia/dysaesthesia (an unpleasant sensation that may occur spontaneously or following stimulation) – Decreased anxiety
2. 6–12 Rx on autonomic region of spine	**2. Acupuncture points**
3. 6–12 Rx on hands and feet	MDC current either
Effects:	– on acupuncture points – around acupuncture needles – attached to acupuncture needles
The above 2 general treatments may have influences on pain, inflammation, immune systems, homeostatic mechanisms, and other systems at present unknown	*Effects:*
	– As above, including stimulation of the meridians – Enhancement of pain relief and mobility
4. General limb	
Effects:	
– Improved circulation – Relief of pain – Decreased swelling – Improvement of the skin and soft tissue as in trauma, burns, and autonomic symptoms	

Different Types of Pain that Respond to MDC

ACUTE—NOCICEPTIVE	CHRONIC—NEUROPATHIC
Local	Local
Referred	Referred
Trigger point (TP)	TP (primary)
Dermatomal	TP (secondary)
	Dermatomal

Treatment of Various Symptoms with MDC

Treatment of Pain/Inflammation

DISEASE	AREA	SIZE OF AFFECTED AREA	DURATION OF Rx	NO. OF Rx
OA, RA, other type of arthritis	Joint	Small/medium	4–8 mins	6 daily or alternate days; then 6 at 1x or 2x weekly; then 1x or 2x monthly
		Large	8–16 mins	6–12 as above
Ankylosing spondylitis	Joint	Medium	4–8 mins	6–12 as above
	SIJ	Large	8–16 mins	6–12 as above
	Spinal	CS–sacrum	16 mins	6–12 as above
		T1–L5	16 mins	6–12 as above
Osteoporosis	Spinal	CS–sacrum	16 mins 1–2x*	6–12 as above
		T1–L5	16 mins 1–2x*	
	Local bone	As for small/medium/large	As above	6–12 as above
Gout	Joint	Small/medium	8 mins	1–3/6 (if resolution has not occurred after 3 treatments, continue for at least 6 treatments)
Posttrauma tear, sprain	Muscle/ligament/tendon	Small, e.g., hand/foot	8 mins	1–3/6
		Large, e.g., calf/thigh/shoulder/spinal	8–16 mins	3–6
Fracture	Bone, peripheral/spinal	Small	6 mins	6
			16 mins 1–2x *	6–8
Neural compression	Spinal	Local joint + dermatomal	16 mins	6–12
	Peripheral, as in CRPS	Spinal—autonomic and/or somatic	16 mins	6–12
		and/or local superior/inferior	8–16 mins	6–12
		Local superior—inferior and/or local	8 mins	3–6/12 (if resolution has not occurred after 6 treatments, continue for at least 12 treatments)

Remarks: 6 or more treatments, either local or peripheral, will produce general effects in the body, resulting from clinically relevant increases in levels of melatonin, leu-enkephalin, beta-endorphins, and adenosine.

Continued maintenance could be considered for chronic disease.

Joints: Small = wrist/ankle; medium = shoulder/elbow/knee; large = hip/SIJ/spinal.

*Severe pain: 16 mins for 1 or 2 Rx with a 5–10 min rest period between treatments.

Treatment of Decreased Mobility/Stiffness

DISEASE	AREA, SIZE	DURATION OF Rx	NO. OF Rx
Any inflammatory joint	Small/medium	8 mins	6–8
	Large	8–16 mins	6–8
Trauma—postinjury muscular, soft tissues	Small/medium	8 mins	3–6
	Large (includes spine)	8–16 mins	3–6
Trauma—postfracture healing period	Small/medium	8 mins	1–3
	Large	8–16 mins	1–6
Neuropathic	Spinal, autonomic and/or somatic	8–16 mins	6+
	Local superior/inferior	8 mins	3–6
	Local	8 mins	3–6

Remarks: Stiffness starts to resolve after the second treatment and is usually measurable even after the first treatment. Some patients respond to one treatment.

Treatment of Swelling/Edema (Including Bruising)

DISEASE	AREA, SIZE	DURATION OF Rx	NO. OF Rx
Any joint, excluding hemarthrosis			
Acute (soft)	Small/medium	8–16 mins	1–6
	Large	8–16 mins	1–6
Chronic (indurated)	Small/medium/large (see also circulation)	16 mins	6–12 daily or alternating days; 2x weekly; 1x weekly; 1–2x monthly
Trauma	Small/medium	8–16 mins	1–3
	Large	16 mins	1–6

Remarks: It is beneficial to include the general circulation in the region or limb in order to obtain the best results (see "Treatment of Circulation Problems" on the next page). Circulatory treatment for chronic edema and poor circulation may require treatment over many months.

Treatment of Circulation Problems

DISEASE	AREA, SIZE	DURATION OF Rx	NO. OF Rx
Venous congestion			
Bilateral limb	Abdominal iliac vessels to plantar surface of feet and/or level of lumbar 2 to plantar surface of feet	16 mins	6–12
Unilateral limb	Abdominal iliac vessel and lumbar 2 to the distal limb surfaces	16 mins	6–12
Trauma	Local region	8–16 mins	1–3
	General limb (see placement of electrodes, page 205)	16 mins	1–6
Neuropathic			
Cold limb	Spinal, autonomic + somatic	16 mins	1–6
	General limb (unilateral or bilateral)	16 mins	1–6
	Local region	8 mins	1–6
Diabetic	Peripheral nerve to distal limb surfaces	8–16 mins	1–6
Central neuropathic or venous	Palmar/plantar surface of hands/feet	16 mins	1–12
Bilateral (usually)	Hands and feet	16 mins	1–12
Joint arthrosis with fluid retention	Spinal, autonomic + somatic	16 mins	1–12
	General limb (unilateral or bilateral)	16 mins	1–12
	Local region	8 mins	1–6/12 (if resolution has not occurred after 6 treatments, continue for at least 12 treatments)
Soft	*Local*	8 mins	1–6
Hard—cellular	*Local +*	16 mins	1–6/12
	General limb and/or spinal—autonomic and/or somatic	16 mins	1–12

Remarks: Any circulatory problem, even if local, will improve with general limb treatment. Circulatory treatment for chronic edema and poor circulation should continue over many months. Changes in size, color, and pain will be observed.

Treatment of Infection

DISEASE	AREA, SIZE	DURATION OF Rx	NO. OF Rx
Local-region wounds, burns	Skin	4–8 mins	1–6
Sinus	Facial	8 mins	1–4
Post-herpetic	Any region; treat spinal, autonomic, and/or somatic first	8 mins	1–6
Damage resulting from infection, e.g., vocal cords, chest	Local region	8 mins	1–4/6 (if resolution has not occurred after 4 treatments, continue for at least 6 treatments)

Remarks: If exacerbation occurs at spinal area or proximal to the regional area of treatment, do not proceed with treatment of the local area.

If a patient improves after first treatment of 4 mins, then possibly increase treatment duration to 8 mins to increase the effects of treatment.

Placement of Electrodes

The following diagrams illustrate where to place electrodes for treatment of various conditions. Trying some of these treatments will indicate the value of MDC therapy as another tool in the armamentarium of the therapist and as another device that a patient may wish to investigate for pain relief.

KEY: READ ALL AS FOLLOWS:

$\boxed{-}$ Electrodes marked as negative polarity

$\boxed{+}$ Electrodes marked as positive polarity

The following symbols are used in pairs: $\boxed{-}\boxed{+}$ $\ominus\oplus$ $\Diamond\Diamond$

Different symbols used in the same diagram indicate different areas of treatment.

C2 This symbol indicates the spinal levels.

The preferred distance between the $\boxed{+}$ and $\boxed{-}$ electrodes is 250 mm on the same plane only. This is with the exception of the face. The eye, nose, and mouth provide sufficient resistance to permit closer proximity of the $\boxed{+}$ and $\boxed{-}$ electrodes.

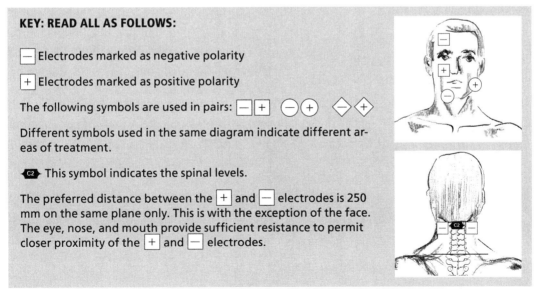

Sinus 1

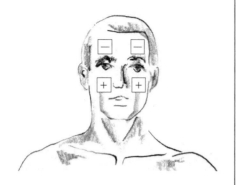

Anteriorly

- ⊟ Frontal sinus bilaterally
- ⊞ Maxillary sinus bilaterally

If maxillary sinus is specifically indicated, reverse the polarity.

Temporomandibular Joint

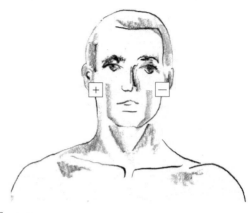

- ⊟ Unilateral temporomandibular joint pain
- ⊞ Indifferent electrode

Sinus 2

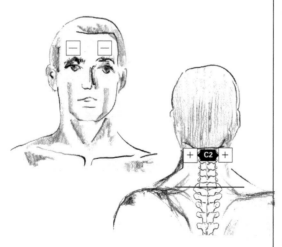

- ⊞ Posteriorly at C2 bilaterally
- ⊟ Anteriorly, frontal sinus bilaterally

Mouth or Cheek

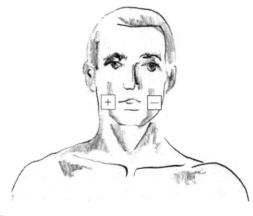

- ⊟ Mouth
- or ⎱ Pain or swelling
- ⊞ Cheek ⎰

Cervical Headache

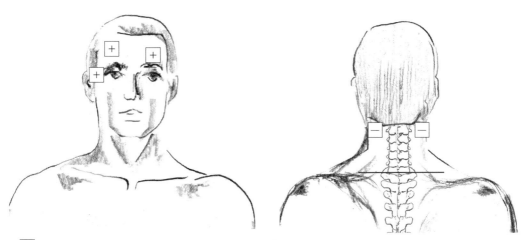

$-$	Unilaterally or bilaterally, slightly lateral to C2
$+$	1) Temporal region
$+$	2) Lateral to outer canthus
$+$	3) Frontalis muscle

Cervical Pain—Trapezius Muscle Spasm

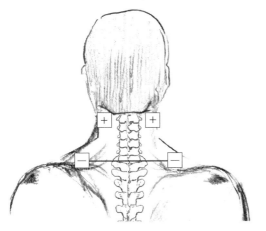

$+$	Occipital nerve
$-$	Upper trapezius bilaterally

Cervical Spondylosis

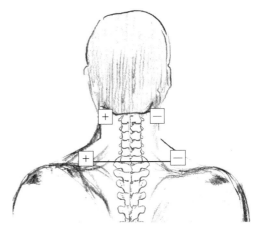

If most pain is on the right cervical spine

$-$	Right trapezuis/scalene muscle spasm
$+$	Indifferent electrode

Cervical Nerve Root Compression

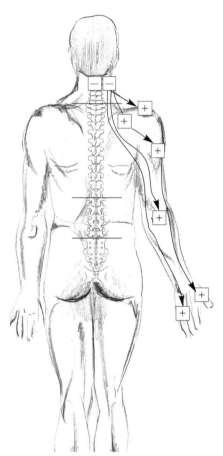

If there is nerve root compression, then the $\boxed{-}$ can be placed centrally on spinous process and on the facet joint at the correct level, and the $\boxed{+}$ can be placed on referring sites:

$\boxed{+}$ can be placed on infraspinatus or supraspinatus muscle

    or   elbow joint
    or   radial nerve
    or   ulnar nerve
    or   outer 2 digits
    or   thumb

Shoulder Pain in Supraspinatus Tendonitis

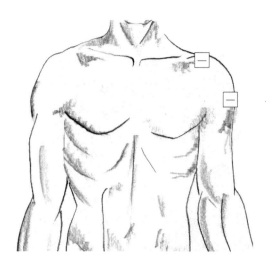

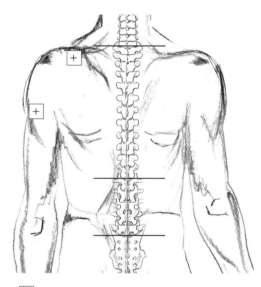

$\boxed{-}$ Anterior: supraspinatus tendon

$\boxed{+}$ Posterior: supraspinatus muscle

Pain in Frozen Shoulder

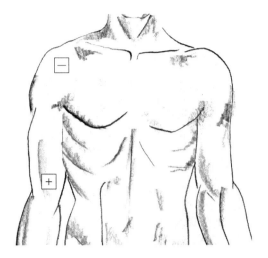

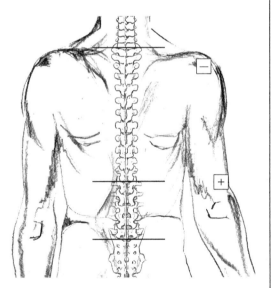

	Anterior and posterior capsule of shoulder joint
+	Pain/muscle spasm

Fracture of the Clavicle, Tear in the Pectoralis Muscle

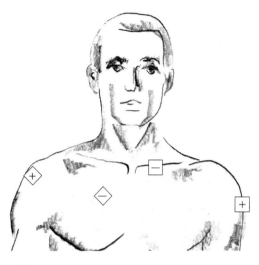

	Fracture of clavicle
+	Indifferent electrode
◇	Tear in pectoralis muscle
◇+	Indifferent electrode

Olecranon Bursitis or OA/RA Wrist

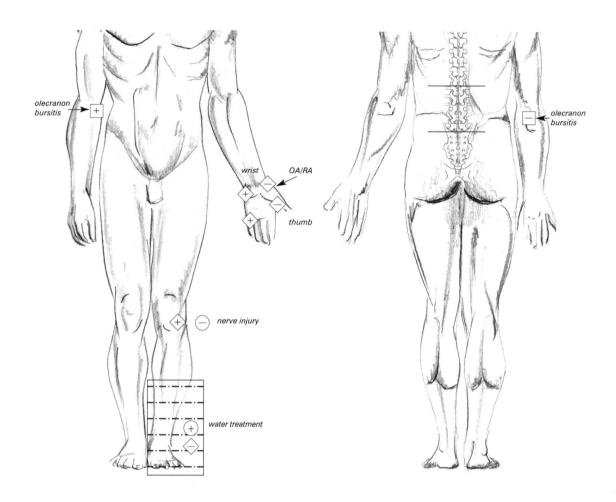

Olecranon bursitis: Place ⊟ on the painful site and ⊞ opposite.

OA/RA wrist: Place ◇⊟ on painful joint and ◇⊞ on opposite side.

If water treatment for hands and/or feet: Place the indifferent on the nerve supply ◇⊞ and the other ◇⊟ freely in the water surrounding the painful joint or on the foot.

Reverse polarity if painful hand or foot is due to "nerve injury"; then ⊟ is placed on nerve supply and ⊞ around the painful hand or foot.

Thoracic Girdle—Pain or Injury

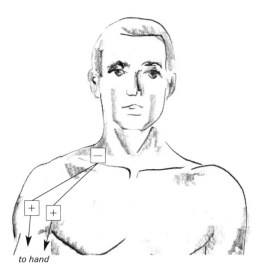

to hand

−	Brachial plexus/cervical spine C7 or thoracic outlet
+	Referred pain in the arm

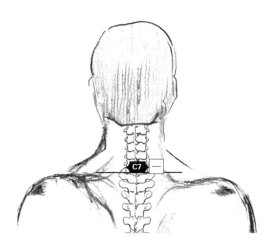

"General Effects" or General "Back Pain"

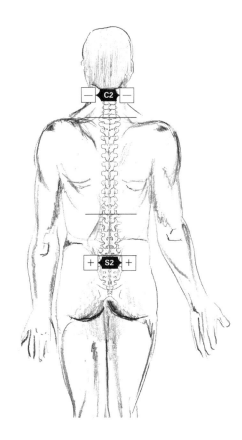

General effects obtained by treatment of the spine from C2 to S1

or

Bilateral hands and feet

or

General back pain with most pain in the upper spinal region. Reverse polarities if pain is localized to the low back.

Note: This treatment may also be used for osteoporosis or ankylosing spondylitis.

Lumbar Inflammatory Joint Pain: 1

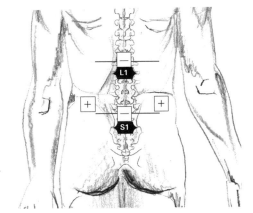

☐ (−) Negative electrode centrally over pain.

☐ (+) Positive electrode bilaterally on quadratus lumborum region

Lumbar Inflammatory Joint Pain: 2

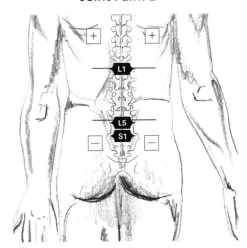

☐ (−) General back pain at L5/S1

☐ (+) Thoracic levels include treatment of the ANS for this region

Note: This treatment may be used for osteoporosis.

Unilateral Lumbar Pain: 1

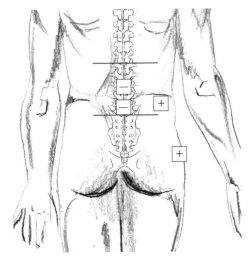

☐ (−) Centrally for L4/5

☐ (+) Unilaterally on the trigger point or area of referred pain

Unilateral Lumbar Pain: 2

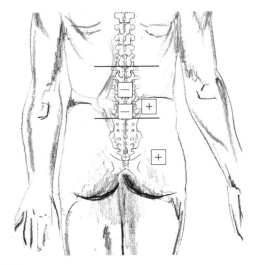

☐ (−) Centrally for L5/S1

☐ (+) Unilaterally on the trigger point or area of referred pain

Circulation to One Leg

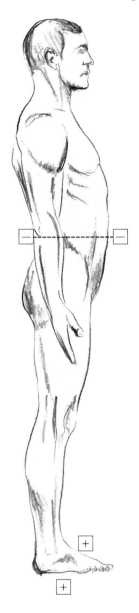

−	Lateral to L2
−	Lateral to umbilicus
+	Dorsum of foot
+	Plantar surface of foot

Circulation to Both Legs

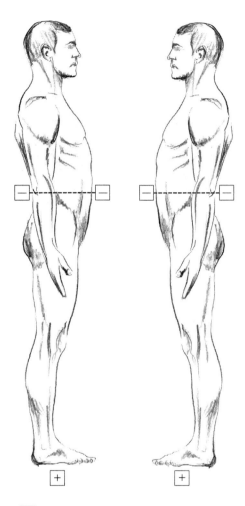

−	Bilaterally to L2 or umbilicus
+	Bilaterally under plantar surface of both feet

Lumbar Nerve Root Compression (NRC): 1

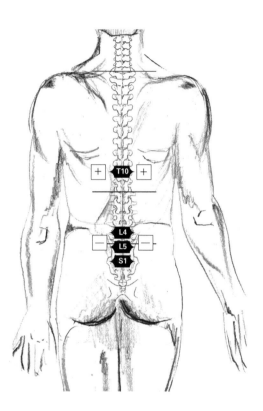

In a NRC, treat the L4–S1 area separately from the referred pain.

$\boxed{-}$ L4–S1 (region of pain)

$\boxed{+}$ T10 (SNS supply to the lumbar region)

Lumbar Nerve Root Compression (NRC): 2

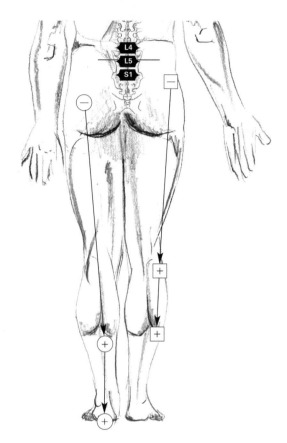

Treat the referred pain with the $\boxed{-}$ electrode on the tender trigger points usually found in the buttock and the $\boxed{+}$ electrode on points of referral in the limb.

$\boxed{-}$ Trigger point in lateral buttock

$\boxed{+}$ Points of referral in the limb for NRC at L4/5

$\ominus$ Trigger point in buttock

$\oplus$ Points of referral in the limb for NRC at L5/S1

Suggested Approach to Multiple Sclerosis: 1

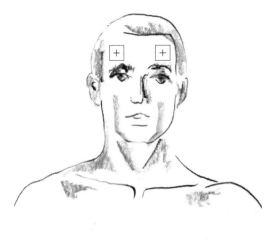

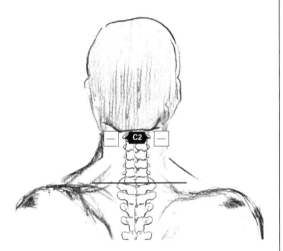

$\boxed{-}$ Stimulation of neural supply from C2 bilaterally

$\boxed{+}$ Stimulation of neural supply to frontal region

Duration: 8 mins
Intensity: 0.9 mA maximum

Suggested Approach to Multiple Sclerosis: 2

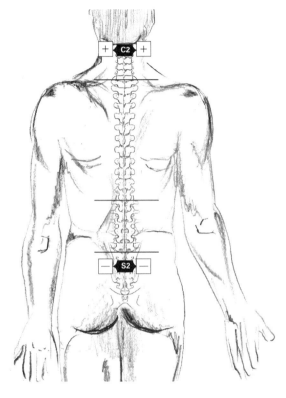

$\boxed{+}$ Stimulation of neural supply at C2 bilaterally

$\boxed{-}$ Stimulation of neural supply at S2 bilaterally

Duration: 16 mins
Intensity: 1+ mA

Reverse polarity if maximal pain is present in the upper spine.

Hip Pain: 1

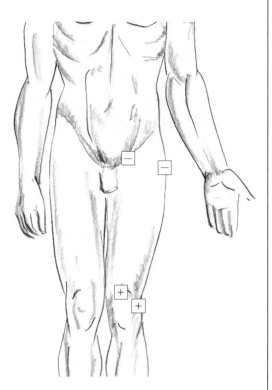

☐ ⊟	Hip joint
☐ ⊞	Hip pain producing referred leg/thigh/knee pain

Hip Pain: 2

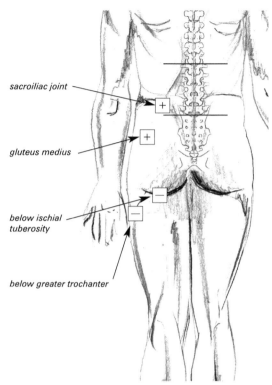

sacroiliac joint

gluteus medius

below ischial tuberosity

below greater trochanter

☐ ⊞	Gluteus medius and sacroiliac joint
☐ ⊟	Hip joint pain producing mostly posterior pain

Hip Pain: 3

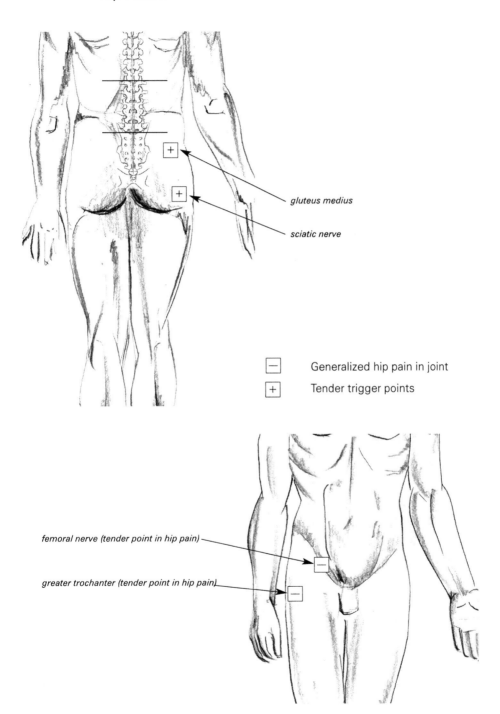

gluteus medius

sciatic nerve

	Generalized hip pain in joint
−	
+	Tender trigger points

femoral nerve (tender point in hip pain)

greater trochanter (tender point in hip pain)

Knee Joint Arthritis: 1

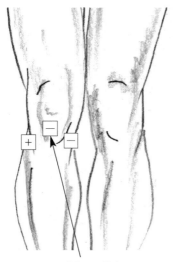

patellofemoral joint

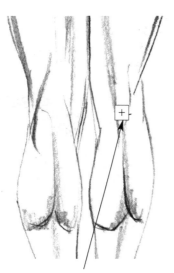

popliteal fossa

−	Patellofemoral joint
−	Medial joint line
+	Popliteal fossa
+	Lateral joint line

Knee Joint Arthritis: 2

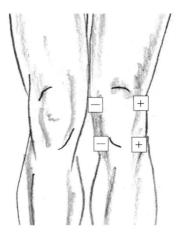

Medial joint lines
or

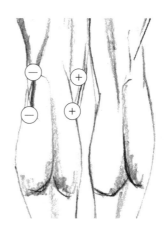

Lateral joint lines

Depending on which joint line has the most pain

−	Pain medial joint line
+	Indifferent electrode
−	Pain lateral joint line
+	Indifferent electrode

Knee Joint Swelling: 1

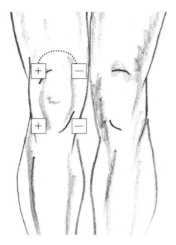

If most of the swelling is medial, place:

2 $-$ medial and

2 $+$ lateral

or vice versa if swelling is lateral.

Knee Joint Swelling: 2

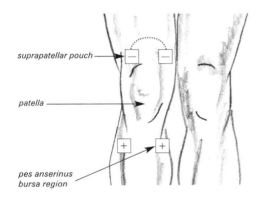

suprapatellar pouch

patella

pes anserinus
bursa region

2 $-$ superiorly below or above suprapatellar pouch

and 2 $+$ below pes anserinus bursa
or below swelling

Recommended Treatment for Osteoarthritis of the Knee

For inflammation, pain, and improvement of range of movement:
Treat the local area for 8 mins:

Daily for first 2 weeks

Alternating days for next 2 weeks

Twice weekly for the next 2 weeks

Once weekly for the next 4 weeks

Once in 2 weeks

Once in 3 weeks

Once monthly (for maintenance,
   if necessary)

Treat for general effects (spinal):

6 treatments consecutively or on
   alternate days, 8–16 mins

Rest treatment for 2 weeks

Repeat 6 treatments as above, if pain
   levels are still high

The general treatment can be given concomitantly with the local treatment.

If pain ceases and mobility improves, treatment may be discontinued at any stage based on the decision of the practitioner or patient.

For swelling, treat for 16 mins:

As above and include the whole leg, but continue once monthly over a protracted period (1 year)

Achilles Tendonitis, Lateral Collateral Ligament (LCL) Sprain

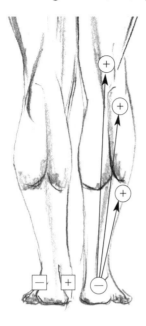

Achilles Tendonitis, Calcaneal Spur

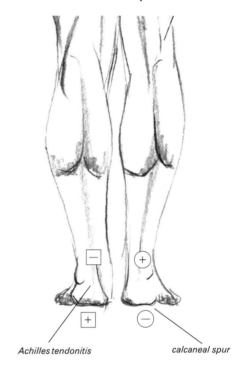

Achilles tendonitis   *calcaneal spur*

LCL SPRAIN

Place ⊟ on LCL and ⊞ on any region opposite

ACHILLES TENDONITIS

⊖ on Achilles tendon and ⊕ on the part of the muscle that has a trigger point

This could be the medial or lateral gastrocnemius, medial or lateral soleus, or sciatic nerve.

☐ ACHILLES TENDONITIS

○ CALCANEAL SPUR

◆ ◆ ◆

These guidelines may also be used for TENS treatment, but TENS may elicit different effects, mostly pain relieving. The treatment protocols that are depicted in the diagrams may assist therapists and patients in the use of many other types of therapy.

ENDNOTES

Chapter 1

1. Fillingim, R.B., "Sex Differences in Analgesic Responses: Evidence from Experimental Pain Models," *European Journal of Anaesthesiology* 19 (2002), suppl. 26: 6–24.

2. Lecture, World Institute of Pain Congress, Tenerife, Canary Islands, Spain, 1999.

3. Carr, D.J., "The Role of Endogenous Opioids and Their Receptors in the Immune System," *Proceedings of the Society for Experimental Biology and Medicine* 198:710–720, http://www.ebmonline.org/cgi/content/abstract/198/2/710.

4. McEwen, B.S., "Protective and Damaging Effects of Stress Mediators," *New England Journal of Medicine* 338 (1998): 171–79.

5. Mersky, H., and N. Bogduk, *Classification of Chronic Pain*, vol. 2 (Seattle, WA: IASP Press, 1994), 41–42, 210–12.

6. Sarno, J.E., *Mind over Back Pain* (New York: Berkeley Publishing Group, 1984); *Healing Back Pain* (New York: Warner Books, 1991); *The Mindbody Prescription* (New York: Warner Books, 1999).

7. Cahill, L., B. Prins, M. Weber, and J.L. McGaugh, "Beta-Adrenergic Activation and Memory for Emotional Events," *Nature* 371 (1994): 702–4.

8. Okifuji, A., E. Fernandez, and J.W. Burns, Workshop on Anger and Pain, IASP Congress, San Diego, CA, 2002.

9. Ibid.

10. Ibid.

11. Harrison, S., and P. Geppetti, "Substance P," *International Journal of Biochemistry and Cell Biology* 33 (2001), 555–76.

12. Kato, Y., C.J. Kowalski, and C.S. Stohler, "Habituation of the Early Pain-Specific Respiratory Response in Sustained Pain," *Pain* 91 (2001): 57–33

13. Jackson, M., *Pain: The Fifth Vital Sign—The Science and Culture of Why We Hurt* (New York: Crown Publishers, 2002).

14. Ibid.

Chapter 2

1. Sarno, J.E., *Mind over Back Pain* (New York: Berkeley Publishing Group, 1984); *Healing Back Pain* (New York: Warner Books, 1991); *The Mindbody Prescription* (New York: Warner Books, 1999).

2. McEwen, B., with E. Lasley, *The End of Stress as We Know It* (Washington, DC: National Academies Press, 2002).

3. "The Science of Stress," from website http://faculty.weber.edu/molpin/healthclasses/1110/bookchapters/stressphysiologychapter.htm. (accessed November 2005).

4. Funes, M. *Laughing Matters* (Dublin, Ireland: Gill and MacMillan, 2000), 33.

5. Gifford, L., "Whiplash Science and Management: Fear Avoidance Beliefs and Behaviour," in *Physiotherapy Pain Association Yearbook 1998–1999: Topical Issues in Pain*, ed. L. Gifford (Falmouth, U.K.: NOI Press, 1998).

Endnotes

Chapter 3

1. Reilly, David. "Enhancing human healing" (editorial), *British Medical Journal* 322 (2001): 120–121.

2. Charon, R., "Narrative, Pain, and Suffering," in *Progress in Pain Research and Management*, vol. 34, ed. D.B. Carr, J.D. Loeser, and D.B. Morris (Seattle: IASP Press, 2005).

3. Charon R., *Narrative Medicine: Honoring the Stories of Illness* (New York: Oxford University Press, 2006).

4. Sluka, K.A., K. Hoeger, and D.A. Skyba, "Basic Science Mechanisms of Nonpharmacological Treatments for Pain: An Updated Review," in *Refresher Course Syllabus*, ed. M.A. Giamberardino, presented at IASP Congress, San Diego, 2002.

5. Goldfarb et al., 1997, cited in Sluka et al., 189.

6. Loeser et al., 2001, cited in Sluka et al., 189.

7. Haier et al., 1981, cited in Sluka et al., 189.

8. Droste et al., 1991, cited in Sluka et al., 189.

9. Lundberg, T., "Is There a Physiological Basis for the Use of Acupuncture in Pain?" Plenary lecture presented at First International Medical Congress on Acupuncture, Barcelona, Spain, 2003.

10. Koltyn, 2000, cited in Sluka et al., 189.

11. Ransford, 1982, cited in Sluka et al., 190.

12. Nutter, 1988, Simons and Birkimer, 1988, cited in Sluka et al., 190.

13. Gurevich et al., 1994, Ferrell, et al., 1997, cited in Sluka et al., 190.

14. Bokun, B., *Humour Therapy* (London: Vita Books, 1986).

15. Berk, L., "PsychoNeuroImmunology Research Society Meetings, 18 April 1996, Santa Monica, California" in *Laughing Matters*, Maria Funes (Dublin, Ireland: Gill and Macmillan Ltd., 2000), 31.

16. Funes, M., 33–34.

17. Ibid.

18. Kato, Y., Kowalski, C.J., and Stohler, C.S., "Habituation of the Early Pain-Specific Respiratory Response in Sustained Pain," *Pain* 91 (2001), 57–63.

19. Benson, H., and M.Z. Klipper, *The Relaxation Response* (New York: Harper Torch, 2000), 9.

20. Benson and Klipper, 38–39.

21. Benson and Klipper, 124–25.

22. Gundel, H., and T.R. Tolle, "How Physical Pain May Interact with Psychological Pain: Evidence for a Mutual Neurobiological Basis of Emotions and Pain," in *Narrative, Pain and Suffering: Progress in Pain Research and Management*, vol. 34, eds. D.B. Carr, J.D. Loeser, and D.B. Morris (Seattle, WA: IASP Press, 2005), 93.

23. Gold, L., "Pain Relief Through Movement Education (Sensory-Motor Integration): Explaining Hanna Somatic Education," http://somatics.com/movement.htm (accessed 19 March 2006).

Chapter 4

1. Shapiro, A.K., and E. Shapiro, "The Powerful Placebo," in *Physiotherapy Pain Association Yearbook 1998–1999: Topical Issues of Pain*, ed. L. Gifford (Falmouth, U.K.: NOI Press, 1998), 11.

2. Wall, P.D., *Pain: The Science of Suffering* (London: Weidenfeld and Nicolson, Orion Publishing Group, 1999), 128.

3. Butler, D., "Integrating Pain Awareness into Physiotherapy: Wise Action for the Future," in *Physiotherapy Pain Association Yearbook 1998–1999: Topical Issues of Pain*, ed. L. Gifford (Falmouth, U.K.: NOI Press, 1998), 12.

4. Benson, H., *The Relaxation Response* (New York: Harper Torch, 2000) 20–21.

5. Wall, 136–38.

6. Berger, P., and L. Matzner, "Study on Osteoarthritis of the Knee Comparing the Effects of APS

Current Therapy with TENS and Placebo," *South African Journal of Anaesthesiology and Analgesia* 5 (1999): 26–39.

7. Pollo, A., M. Amanzio, A. Arslanian, C. Casadio, G. Maggi, and F. Benedetti, "Response Expectancies in Placebo Analgesia and Their Clinical Relevance," *Pain* 93 (2001): 77–84.

8. Amanzio, M., A. Pollo, G. Maggi, and F. Benedetti, "Response Variability to Analgesics: A Role for Non-Specific Activation of Endogenous Opioids," *Pain* 90 (2001): 205–15.

9. Wall, 128.

10. Price, D.D., L.S. Milling, I. Kirsh, A. Duff, G.H. Montgomery, and S.S. Nicholl, "An Analysis of Factors that Contribute to the Magnitude of Placebo Analgesia," *Pain* 83 (1999): 147–56.

11. Butler, 11.

12. Fields, H., "Reward Expectancy and the Biology of Placebo Analgesia," lecture at the 11th IASP Congress, Sydney, 2005.

13. Dossey, L., *Healing Words: The Power of Prayer and the Practice of Medicine* (New York: HarperCollins, 1993).

14. Khalsa, Dharma Singh, and Cameron Stauth, *Meditation as Medicine* (New York: Pocket Books, 2001), 126–27.

15. Benson, H., *Timeless Healing: The Power and Biology of Belief* (New York: Scribner, 1996), 12.

16. Cane, W., *The Art of Hugging* (New York: St. Martin's Griffin, 1996).

17. Montagu, A., *Touching: The Human Significance of the Skin* (New York: Columbia University Press, 1971).

18. Hanneman, H., "Magnetic Therapy," 1990, http://health.groups.yahoo.com/group/Lyon Legacy/message/1 (accessed November 2005).

19. Norris, N.C., *The Book of Magnetic Healing and Treatments* (Victoria, Australia: International Research and Development Magnetic Health Products Organization, 1995), 9.

20. Hannemann, H., *Magnet Therapy: Balancing Your Body's Energy Flow for Self-Healing* (New York: Sterling, 1990).

21. Research by K. Nakagawa, M.D. See, for example, "Magnetic Therapy," www.painxequine.com/mag_therapy.htm (accessed 19 March 2006).

22. Research by P. Kokoschinegg. See, for example, "Magnetic Wound Treatment Externally Applied Magnetic Fields," www.worldofmagnets.co.uk/articles/wound.htm (accessed 19 March 2006).

23. Norris.

24. Mitchell, R., clinical studies on magnets and energy healing since the 1980s, and articles published in *Meridian,* newsletter of the Acupuncture Association of the South African Society of Physiotherapy.

25. Karu, T.L., "Photobiological Fundamentals of Low-Power Laser Therapy," *IEEE Journal of Quantum Electronics* QE23 10 (1987): 1703–17.

26. Meister, E., A.E. Meister, and A. Meister, "The Biomedical Effect of Laser Application," *Lasers in Surgery and Medicine* 5 (1985): 31–39.

27. Gamaleya, N.F., "Laser Biomedical Research," in *Tae-MSSR Laser Applications in Medicine and Biology* (New York: Plenum Press, 1977).

28. Pascoe, P.J., "Alternative Therapies for Pain Management," *Journal of the American Veterinary Medical Association* 221:6 (2002), 779–780.

29. Merrell, W.C., and E. Shalts, "Homeopathy," *Medical Clinics of North America* 86 (2002): 47–61.

30. Kleinjnen, J., P. Knipschild, and G. ter Riet, "Clinical Trials of Homeopathy," *British Medical Journal* 302 (1991): 316–23; Linde, K., et al., "Are the Clinical Effects of Homeopathy Placebo Effects?

A Meta-Analysis of Placebo-Controlled Trials," *Lancet* 350 (1997): 834–43; http://www.healingchron icpain.org/content/introduction/comp_home.asp (accessed 2005).

Chapter 5

1. Melzack, R., "The McGill Pain Questionnaire," *Pain* 1 (1975): 275–77.

2. Bokun, B., *Humour Therapy* (London: Veritas Foundation Press, 1986), 16.

Chapter 7

1. Chan, S.H., "What Is Being Stimulated in Acupuncture? Evaluation of the Existence of a Specific Substrate," *Neuroscience Biobehavioural Review* 8 (1984), 25–33, cited in Yun-Tao Ma, Mila Ma, and Zang Hee Cho, *Biomedical Acupuncture for Pain Management: An Integrative Approach* (St. Louis, MO: Elsevier, 2005), 1.

2. Helms, J.M., *Acupuncture Energetics: A Clinical Approach for Physicians* (Berkeley, CA: Medical Acupuncture Publishers, 1995), 20–21.

3. Tin Yau So, J., *The Book of Acupuncture Points* (Brookline, MA: Paradigm Publications, 1985).

4. The sources for much of the information in this section are: Ma, Ma, and Cho, 1–35; and Helms, 32–41.

5. Han, J.S., ed., *The Neurochemical Basis of Pain Relief by Acupuncture: A Collection of Papers 1973–1987* (Beijing, China: Beijing Medical University, 1987).

6. Lundberg, T., "Is There a Physiological Basis for the Use of Acupuncture in Pain?" Plenary lecture, First International Medical Congress on Acupuncture, Barcelona, Spain, 2003.

7. Han, J.S., "Footsteps on the Neurochemical Study of Acupuncture Analgesia," first published in *Chinese Journal of Integrated Traditional and Western Medicine* 6 (1986), reprinted in Han, *The Neurochemical Basis of Pain Relief by Acupuncture.*

8. Many such studies exist; I've listed only a small sampling of literature here: (1) Han, J.S., "Physiologic and Neurochemical Basis of Acupuncture Analgesia," first published in *The International Textbook of Cardiology*, Cheng, T.O., ed. (New York: Pergamon, 1986), 1124–32, reprinted in Han, *The Neurochemical Basis of Pain Relief by Acupuncture*; (2) Cho, Z.H., E.K. Wong, and J. Fallon, *Neuro-Acupuncture: Scientific Evidence of Acupuncture Revealed* (Los Angeles, CA: Q-Puncture Inc., 2001). Z.H. Cho is affiliated with the Department of Radiological Sciences and Psychiatry and Human Behavior, University of California, Irvine.

9. Brinkhaus, B., et al., "Acupuncture Randomized Trials (ART) in Patients with Chronic Low Back Pain and Osteoarthritis of the Knee: Design and Protocols," *Forsch Komplementärmed Klass Naturheilkd* 10:4 (Aug. 2003): 185–91; Melchart, D., et al., "Acupuncture Randomized Trials (ART) in Patients with Migraine or Tension-Type Headache: Design and Protocols," *Forsch Komplementärmed Klass Naturheilkd* 10:4 (Aug. 2003): 179–84.

10. Zhang, Y., *ECIWO Biology and Medicine: A New Theory of Conquering Cancer and a Completely New Acupuncture Therapy* (People's Republic of China, Huehaote, Neimenggu: Neimenggu People's Press (Publisher), 1987), 5.

11. According to S.L. Rosenblatt, former president of the California Acupuncture College, this proverb was included in Tin Yau So's *The Book of Acupuncture Points* (see note 3). Rosenblatt calls Dr. Tin Yau So the "father of American acupuncture."

12. Peilin, S., ed. *The Treatment of Pain with Chinese Herbs and Acupuncture* (Edinburgh, U.K.: Churchill Livingstone, Harcourt Publishers, 2002). Peilin is a professor of medicine at Guangxi College of TCM and Jiangxi College of TCM, in China, and a professor of TCM at Jing Ming College of Oriental Medicine, in Belgium.

Chapter 8

1. Becker, R.O., "The Role of the Orthopaedic Surgeon in the Development of Bioconductivity," *Journal of Bioconductivity* 2 (1983): 1.

2. Cheng, N., et al., "The Effects of Electrical Currents on ATP Generation, Protein Synthesis and Membrane Transport in Rat Skin," *Clinical Orthopaedics* 171 (1982): 264–72.

3. Seegers, J.C., C.A. Engelbrecht, and D.H. van Papendorp, "Activation of Signal-Transduction Mechanisms May Underlie the Therapeutic Effects of an Applied Electric Field," *Medical Hypotheses* 57 (2001): 224–30.

4. Low, J., and A. Reed, "Electrical Stimulation of Nerve and Muscle," in *Electrotherapy Explained*, 2d ed. (Oxford, England: Butterworth Heinmann, 1995), 43–100.

5. Additional sources for this section are: Seegers, J.C., et al., "A Pulsed DC Electric Field Affects P2-Purinergic Receptor Functions by Altering the ATP Levels in In Vitro and In Vivo Systems," *Medical Hypotheses* 58 (2002): 171–76; and Seegers et al., 2001.

6. Becker, R.O., and G. Selden, *The Body Electric* (New York: William Morrow & Co., 1985).

7. Melzack, R., and P.D. Wall, "Pain Mechanisms: A New Theory," *Science* 150 (1965): 971–78.

8. Woolf, C.J., and J.W. Thompson, "Stimulation-Induced Analgesia: Transcutaneous Electrical Nerve Stimulation (TENS) and Vibration," in *Textbook of Pain*, 3rd ed., eds. P.D. Wall, and R. Melzack (Edinburgh, U.K.: Churchill, Livingstone, 1995), 1205.

9. Berger, P., "The Role of the Physiotherapist in the Treatment of Complex Peripheral Pain Syndromes," *Pain Reviews* 6 (1999): 211–32.

10. Stilz, R.J., H. Carron, and D.B. Sanders, "Reflex Sympathetic Dystrophy in a Six-Year-Old: Successful Treatment by Transcutaneous Electrical Nerve Stimulation," *Anaesthetics and Analgesia* 56 (1977): 438–41.

11. Sluka, K.A., M.K. Hoeger, and D.A. Skyba, *Basic Science Mechanisms of Nonpharmacological Treatments for Pain: An Updated Review*, Refresher Course Syllabus, ed. M.A. Giamberadino (Seattle, WA: IASP Press, 2002), 189–202.

12. Chandran, P., and K.A. Sluka, "The Development of Opioid Tolerance with Repeated Transcutaneous Electrical Nerve Stimulation," *Pain* 102 (2003): 195–201.

13. Munsat, T.L., D. McNeal, and R. Walters, "Effects of Nerve Stimulation on Human Muscle," *Archives of Neurology* 33 (1976): 608.

14. Stannish, W.D., et al., "The Effects of Immobilization and Electrical Stimulation on Muscle Glycogen and Myofibrillar ATPase," *Canadian Journal of Applied Sports Sciences* 7 (1982): 267.

15. Green, D.M., "Clinical Studies on Horses and Humans after Redeveloping and Using the Transeva in Pietermaritzburg Kwa-Zulu Natal, South Africa," (unpublished).

16. Becker, R.O., and G. Selden, *The Body Electric* (New York: Morrow, 1985) cited in M.R. Gersh, *Electrotherapy in Rehabilitation* (Philadelphia, PA: F.A. Davis Company, 1992), 167.

17. Sacks, S.M., and J.A. Ernst, "Retrospective Study of Sympathetic Therapy for Pain Attenuation in 197 Patients," 2001 (unpublished).

18. Berger, P., "Pilot Study on a Trial of Nine Patients with Complex Regional Pain Syndrome to Investigate Pain Attenuation with Sympathetic Therapy," 2001 (unpublished).

Chapter 9

1. Low, J., and A. Reed, "Electrical Stimulation of Nerve and Muscle," in *Electrotherapy Explained*, 2d ed. (Oxford, England: Butterworth Heinemann, 1995), 49.

2. Low and Reed, 99–100.

3. Seegers, J.C., C.A. Engelbrecht, and D.H. Van Papendorp, "Activation of Signal-Transduction Mechanisms May Underlie the Therapeutic Effects of an Applied Electric Field," *Medical Hypotheses* 57 (2001): 224–30.

4. De Wet, E.H., J.M.C. Oosthuizen, C.L. Odendaal, and E.A. Shipton, "Neurochemical Mechanisms that May Underlie the Clinical Efficacy of APS Therapy in Chronic Pain Management," *South African Journal of Anaesthesiology and Analgesia* 5:1 (1999): 33–38.

5. Odendaal, C.L., and G. Joubert, "APS Therapy: A New Way of Treating Chronic Backache—A Pilot Study," *South African Journal of Anaesthesiology and Analgesia* 5:1 (1999): 26–29.

6. Berger, P., and L. Matzner, "Study on Osteoarthritis of the Knee Comparing the Effects of APS Current Therapy with TENS and Placebo," *South African Journal of Anaesthesiology and Analgesia* 5:2 (1999): 26–39.

7. Seegers, et al.

8. For discussion of a few more studies on APS, see Berger, P., *Introducing Action Potential Currents* (Pretoria, South Africa: Art2Print, 1999).

Chapter 10

1. Berger, P., "The Role of the Physiotherapist in the Treatment of Complex Peripheral Pain Syndromes," *Pain Reviews* 6 (1999): 211–32.

2. Stilz, R.J., H. Carron, and D.B. Sanders, "Reflex Sympathetic Dystrophy in a Six-Year-Old: Successful Treatment by Transcutaneous Electrical Nerve Stimulation," *Anaesthetics and Analgesia* 56 (1977) 438–41.

3. Berger, 226.

Chapter 11

1. Prudden, B., *Pain Erasure* (New York: Ballantine, 1985).

2. Kendall, K.P., and E.K. Mc Creary, *Muscle Testing and Function*, 3rd ed. (London: Williams and Wilkins, 1982).

3. McKenzie, R.A., *McKenzie Back Exercises* (Wellington, New Zealand: Wellington Physiotherapy Clinic, 1977).

Chapter 12

1. Urry, H.L., et al., "Making a Life Worth Living: Neural Correlates of Well-Being," *Psychological Science* 15:6 (June 2004): 367–72.

2. Evian, G., *Integrative Neuroscience* (Amsterdam: Harwood Academic Publishers, 2000), 19.

3. Davidson, R.J., et al., "Alterations in Brain and Immune Function," *Psychosomatic Medicine* 65 (2003): 564–70.

4. Kircher, T., *Herbs for the Soul* (London: Thorsons, 2001); Norman, C., *The Illustrated Encyclopedia of Healing Remedies* (London: Element Books, 1998); Roberts, M., *The A–Z of Herbs* (Cape Town, South Africa: Struik Publishers, 1993).

5. Lewandowski, W., M. Good, and C. Burke-Druckner, "Changes in the Meaning of Pain with the Use of Guided Imagery," *Pain Management Nursing* 6 (2005): 58–67.

Appendix A

1. Peilin, S., ed., *The Treatment of Pain with Chinese Herbs and Acupuncture* (London: Churchill Livingstone, 2002), 3.

2. Tin Yau So, J., *The Book of Acupuncture Points: Volume 1 of a Complete Course in Acupuncture* (Brookline, MA: Paradigm Publications, 1984), 1.

3. Filshie, J., et al., "Acupuncture for the Relief of Cancer-Related Breathlessness," *Palliative Medicine* 10 (1996): 145–50.

4. Ellis, N., *Acupuncture in Clinical Practice: A Guide for Health Professionals* (Cheltenham, U.K.: Stanley Thornes, 2000).

5. Wong, J.Y., and L.M. Rapson, "Acupuncture in the Management of Pain of Musculoskeletal and Neurologic Origin," *Complementary Therapies in Physical Medicine and Rehabilitation* 10:3 (1999): 531–45, vii–viii. (Dr. Linda Rapson is Executive President of the Acupuncture Foundation of Canada Institute; she lectures to health-care professionals across Canada and internationally on acupuncture and its integration into Western medicine and physiotherapy.)

6. Tukmachi, E., E. Dumpsey, and R. Jubb, "Acupuncture in Knee Osteoarthritis: A Randomised Controlled Trial," presented at the meeting of the British Medical Acupuncture Society, Bournemouth, U.K., 2001.

7. Broumas, G., et al., "Electroacupuncture for Knee Pain in Elderly Patients," paper presented by the Pain Relief Unit and Anaesthetic Department of the General Hospital, Nikea, Piraeus, Greece, Algos Congress 2002 of the World Institute of Pain meeting, Santorini, Greece, 2002.

8. Wong and Rapson.

9. Wong and Rapson.

10. Wong and Rapson.

11. Yun-Tao Ma, Mila Ma, and Zang Hee Cho, *Biomedical Acupuncture* (St. Louis, MO: Elsevier, 2005).

12. Berger, P., "Combining Ancient Chinese Treatment ('Seven-Star'), Needling, and Cupping with Modern Physiotherapy Relieves Pain, Oedema and Improves Mobility: Four Case Studies," *South African Journal of Anaesthesiology and Analgesia* 6 (2000): 26–31.

13. Chan Gunn, C., *The Gunn Approach to the Treatment of Chronic Pain: Intramuscular Stimulation for Myofascial Pain of Radiculopathic Origin* (London: Churchill Livingstone, 1989).

Appendix B

1. Shealy, C.N., "Transcutaneous Nerve Stimulation for the Control of Pain," *Emergency Medicine* 1 (1974): 6.

GLOSSARY

A-alpha, A-beta, A-delta, C fibers: nerve fibers connected to different types of receptors in the skin, muscle, and internal organs that transmit information about touch and pain to the spinal cord and brain. They come in different diameters and can be divided into different groups based on their size (in order of decreasing size: A-alpha, A-beta, A-delta, and C). A-alpha, A-beta, and A-delta fibers are insulated with myelin. C fibers are unmyelinated. The thickness of the nerve fiber correlates to the speed with which information travels along it—the thicker the fiber, the faster information travels. A-alpha nerve fibers carry information related to proprioception (muscle sense). A-beta nerve fibers carry information related to touch. A-delta nerve fibers carry information related to pain and temperature and are often referred to as thermoreceptors. C nerve fibers carry information related to pain, temperature, and itch.

acetylcholine: a chemical produced in nerve endings that is essential for transmission of nerve impulses.

acupuncture: an original Chinese practice of puncturing the body (as with needles) at specific points to cure disease or relieve pain.

adrenaline/noradrenaline: two separate but related hormones secreted by the medulla of the adrenal glands. They are also produced at the ends of sympathetic nerve fibers, where they serve as chemical mediators for conveying nerve impulses to effector organs (organs that become active in response to stimulation). Chemically, the two compounds differ only slightly, and they exert similar pharmacological actions, which resemble the effects of the flight-or-fight response.

algogenic: pain inducing; something that is painful or that increases pain.

allodynia: when a body part is painful if moved, touched, or vibrated.

allostatis: another word for "homeostasis," a state in which the balance of the body's metabolic activity is kept stable.

amygdala: an almond-shaped set of neurons located deep in the brain; it has been shown to play a key role in the processing of emotions, and forms part of the limbic system. In humans and other animals it is linked to both fear and pleasure responses.

analgesia: pain relief or relief from pain.

autonomic nervous system: sometimes called the involuntary nervous system; consists of the sympathetic and parasympathetic nervous systems. Conveys sensory impulses from the blood vessels, the heart, and all of the organs in the chest, abdomen, and pelvis through nerves to other parts of the brain (mainly the medulla, pons, and hypothalamus). These impulses often do not reach our consciousness, but elicit largely automatic or reflex responses through the efferent (outgoing from the central nervous system) autonomic nerves, thereby triggering appropriate reactions of the heart, vascular system, and other bodily organs to variations in environmental temperature, posture, food intake, stressful experiences, and other changes to which all individuals are exposed. The sympathetic nervous system accelerates heart rate, constricts blood vessels, and raises blood pressure; the parasympathetic nervous system slows heart rate, increases intestinal and glandular activity, and relaxes sphincter muscles.

catecholamine: any of several compounds occurring naturally in the body that serve as hormones or as neurotransmitters in the sympathetic nervous system. The catecholamines include such compounds as epinephrine (adrenaline), norepinephrine, and dopamine. Epinephrine and norepinephrine, which are also hormones, are secreted by the adrenal medulla, and norepinephrine is also secreted by some nerve fibers. These substances prepare the body to meet emergencies such as cold, fatigue, and shock, and norepinephrine is probably a chemical transmitter at nerve synapses.

complex regional pain syndrome (CRPS): a chronic pain condition. The key symptom is continuous, intense pain out of proportion to the severity of the injury, which gets worse rather than better over time. CRPS most often affects one of the arms, legs, hands, or feet. Often the pain spreads to include the entire arm or leg. Typical features include dramatic changes in the color and temperature of the skin over the affected limb or body part, accompanied by intense burning pain, skin sensitivity, sweating, and swelling. Doctors aren't sure what causes CRPS. In some cases the sympathetic nervous system plays an important role in sustaining the pain. Another theory is that CRPS is caused by a triggering of the immune response, which leads to the characteristic inflammatory symptoms of redness, warmth, and swelling in the affected area.

cortisol: a hormone produced by the adrenal glands that helps to regulate blood pressure and cardiovascular function as well as the body's use of proteins, carbohydrates, and fats. Cortisol secretion increases in response to physical and psychological stress during the fight-or-flight response, which is why it is sometimes called the stress hormone.

deafferentation pain: pain due to loss of sensory input into the central nervous system, as occurs, for example, with avulsion (forcible separation or detachment) of the brachial plexus (a network of nerves lying mostly in the armpit and supplying nerves to the chest, shoulder, and arm), or other types of damage to peripheral nerves, or because of pathology of the central nervous system.

electroacupuncture: a procedure quite similar to traditional acupuncture (in that the same points on the body are stimulated) but the needles are attached to a device that generates continuous electric pulses. The frequency and intensity of the impulses are adjusted based on the condition being treated. Electroacupuncture uses two needles at a time so that the impulses can pass from one needle to the other. Several pairs of needles can be stimulated simultaneously. Treatment usually lasts for no longer than 30 minutes per session.

endorphins: endogenous opioid proteins produced by the pituitary gland and the hypothalamus in vertebrates. They resemble the opiates in their abilities to produce analgesia and a sense of well-being. In other words, they work as "natural painkillers."

enkephalin: one of several naturally occurring morphinelike substances (endorphins) released from nerve endings of the central nervous system and the adrenal medulla. They act as analgesics and sedatives in the body and appear to affect mood and motivation.

epidural: an injection into the epidural space of the spinal cord. Scientific studies often demonstrate inflammation of the spinal nerves following prolonged compression, which leads to irritation and swelling. This irritation occurs at the level of the root of the lumbar nerves. The injection of steroids, which are potent anti-inflammatories, is made into the epidural space, close to the affected nerve roots. These injections are given by pain-management specialists who are well trained in this technique. Improvement of the symptoms appears to correlate well with the resolution of the nerve root inflammation. These injections are most effective when given in the first weeks of the onset of pain. Usually, two to three injections, administered one to two weeks apart, are required. Only a single injection is given if complete pain relief is achieved.

femoral/tibial plateau: the femur is the thighbone, the longest bone in the body. The lower end joins the tibia (shin) to form the knee joint. At the lower end of the femur lie two processes called the lateral condyle and the medial condyle. The two condyles slide or rotate along the tibial plateau. The femur also has a patellar groove that acts as a guide for the patella and forms the patellofemoral joint. The tibia is the inner and thicker of the two long bones in the lower leg; also called the shinbone. Its upper end is expanded into medial and lateral condyles that unite with the femoral condyles.

fibromyalgia: a widespread musculoskeletal pain and fatigue disorder for which the cause is still unknown. Fibromyalgia means pain in the muscles, ligaments, and tendons—the body's soft fibrous tissues. Most patients with fibromyalgia report aching throughout the entire body. Their muscles may feel like they have been pulled or overworked. Sometimes the muscles twitch and at other times they burn. More women than men are afflicted with fibromyalgia, and it shows up in people of all ages.

fight-or-flight response: also called the acute stress response; first described by Walter Cannon in 1929. The theory states that animals react to threats with a general discharge of the sympathetic nervous system. The response was later recognized as the first stage of a general adaptation syndrome that regulates stress responses among vertebrates and other organisms. In layman's terms, an animal has two options when faced with danger. It can either face the threat ("fight") or avoid the threat ("flight").

hyperalgesia: an extreme sensitivity to pain that in one form is caused by damage to pain receptors in the body's soft tissues. Hyperalgesia can be experienced in focal, discrete areas, or as a more diffuse, body-wide form. The focal form is typically associated with injury, and is divided into two subtypes: *primary hyperalgesia* describes pain sensitivity that occurs directly in the damaged tissues; *secondary hyperalgesia* describes pain sensitivity that occurs in surrounding undamaged tissues.

hyperesthesia: a neurological symptom involving an unusual increased or altered sensitivity to sensory stimuli.

hypothalamus: located in the brain below the thalamus; functions to regulate certain metabolic processes and other autonomic activities. It links the nervous system to the endocrine system by synthesizing and secreting neurohormones, often called *releasing hormones*, that control the secretion of other hormones.

infrapatellar nerve: a branch of the saphenous nerve that passes downward on the medial side of leg at the lower end of the femur and supplies skin over the medial side and front of the knee and patellar ligament.

meridian: in traditional Chinese medicine, the pathways of positive and negative energy that lie in distinct patterns over the exterior of the body and integrate some of the communication between the various parts of the body. They have been detected by electrical devices that can demonstrate differences in resistance.

motor nerve: an efferent (outgoing from the central nervous system) nerve conveying an impulse that excites muscular contraction. Motor nerves in the autonomic nervous system also elicit secretions from glandular surfaces.

myofascial pain syndromes: pain syndromes that are caused by and are maintained by one or more active trigger points in muscles or tender areas of the soft tissue (fascia) and their associated reflexes.

neuralgia: a painful disorder of the cranial nerves. Under the general heading of neuralgia are trigeminal neuralgia, atypical facial pain, and post-herpetic neuralgia (caused by shingles or herpes). The affected nerves are responsible for sensing touch, temperature, and pressure in the facial area from the jaw to the forehead. The disorder generally causes short episodes (usually lasting less than two minutes) of excruciating pain, and on only one side of the face. Other nerves in the body may also become susceptible to this disorder (e.g., as with diabetic neuropathy).

neuroma: a benign tumor or thickening of nerve tissue.

nocebo effect: an ill effect caused by the suggestion or belief that something is harmful. See also "placebo effect."

nociceptor: a sensory receptor that responds to pain.

noradrenaline: a substance, both hormone and neurotransmitter, secreted by the adrenal medulla and the nerve endings of the sympathetic nervous system to cause vasoconstriction and increases in heart rate, blood pressure, and blood sugar levels.

norepinephrine: see "noradrenaline."

opioid: any agent that binds to the body's opioid receptors, found principally in the central nervous system and gastrointestinal tract. There are four broad classes of opioids: endogenous opioid peptides, produced in the body; opium alkaloids, such as morphine (the prototypical opioid) and codeine; semisynthetic opioids such as heroin and oxycodone; and fully synthetic opioids such as pethidine and methadone that have structures unrelated to the opium alkaloids. These substances, whether endogenous or administered, relieve pain and improve mood.

parasympathetic nervous system: see "autonomic nervous system."

physiotherapy: treatment of disease by physical and mechanical means (as massage, regulated exercise, water, light, heat, electricity, and acupuncture or dry needling).

placebo effect: improvement in a patient's condition that occurs in response to treatment but cannot be considered due to the specific treatment used. The power of suggestion has been credited with creating both pleasant results and harmful ones (nocebo effect). "The physician's belief in the treatment and the patient's faith in the physician exert a mutually reinforcing effect; the result is a powerful remedy that is almost guaranteed to produce an improvement and sometimes a cure."

—Petr Skrabanek and James McCormick, *Follies and Fallacies in Medicine.*

plum-blossom needling: the application of an acupuncture device that looks like a small hammer with seven small needles embedded in its tip. This device is lightly tapped on the skin to produce a reddening or to break the skin to release a few drops of blood. The technique may relieve pain, swelling, and pressure in the tissues under the tapped area.

qi (also spelled *ch'i, chi,* or *ki):* a fundamental concept of everyday Chinese culture, most often defined as "air" or "breath" and, by extension, "life force" or "spiritual energy" that is part of everything that exists. References to qi or similar philosophical concepts as a type of metaphysical energy that sustains living beings are used in many belief systems, especially in Asia. Stimulation of qi in this book refers to the stimulation by acupuncture needles of electrical energy in the area treated.

referred pain: pain from a malfunctioning, diseased area of the body or nerve that is perceived in another area, often far from the origin; often occurs when a nerve in the spine is compressed or squeezed, causing pain down a leg or arm.

relaxation response: activation of the parasympathetic nervous system that causes a decrease in heart and breathing rates and a balancing of the metabolic processes; can be consciously triggered by using relaxation techniques, deep breathing, visualization, and/or meditation.

sensory nerve: an afferent (incoming to the central nervous system) nerve that conveys information from the periphery (skin and outside environment). Sensory nerve impulses are processed by the central nervous system to become part of the organism's perception of self and environment.

substance P: a polypeptide in the central nervous system that has been associated with the regulation of mood disorders, anxiety, stress, reinforcement, neurogenesis, neurotoxicity, nausea/emesis, and pain. It also has effects as a potent vasodilator.

Substance P is involved in the transmission of pain impulses from peripheral receptors to the central nervous system. It has been theorized that it plays a part in fibromyalgia. Capsaicin has been shown to reduce levels of substance P, probably by reducing the number of C-fiber nerves or causing these nerves to be more tolerant.

sympathectomy: a surgical procedure involving cauterization (cutting and sealing) of a portion of the sympathetic nerve chain that runs down the backbone, parallel to the spinal cord. This operation permanently interrupts the nerve signal that causes pain that appears to have sympathetically maintained symptoms.

sympathetic nervous system: see "autonomic nervous system."

thalamus: a structure located in the center of the brain. Functionally, it can be thought of as a relay station for nerve impulses carrying sensory information into the brain. The thalamus receives these sensory inputs as well as inputs from other parts of the brain and determines which of these signals to forward to the cerebral cortex.

transcutaneous electrical nerve stimulation (TENS): electrical current that passes through the skin and stimulates sensory nerves that relay information to the spinal cord and brain; used in the treatment of various pain disorders. The current used in TENS treatment has a specific frequency, pulse width, and alternating current that produces an impulse with no net charge (the negative and positive charges are equal).

Recommended Reading

Alton, J., *Living Qigong: The Chinese Way to Good Health and Long Life* (Boston & London: Shambhala, 1997).

Benson, H., *The Relaxation Response* (New York: Harper Torch, 2000).

Bloom, W., *The Endorphin Effect: A Breakthrough Strategy for Holistic Health and Spiritual Well-being* (London: Judy Piatkus Publishers, 2001).

Bokun, B., *Humour Therapy* (London: Vita Books, 1986).

Butler, D., and Moseley, L., *Explain Pain* (Adelaide, South Australia: Noigroup Publications, 2003).

Cane, W., *The Art of Hugging*, 1st ed. (New York: St. Martin's Griffin, 1996).

Caudill, M.A., *Managing Pain before It Manages You* (New York: Guilford Press, 2002).

Dossey, L., *The Power of Prayer and the Practice of Medicine* (New York: Harper Paperbacks, 1993).

Fumes, M., *Laughing Matters* (Dublin, Ireland: Gill & Macmillan, 2000).

Gifford, L., "Whiplash Science and Management: Fear Avoidance Beliefs and Behaviour," in *Physiotherapy Pain Association Year Book 1998–1999: Topical Issues in Pain*, ed. L. Gifford (Falmouth, U.K.: NOI Press, 1998).

Goleman, D., ed., *Healing Emotions: Conversations with the Dalai Lama on Mindfulness, Emotions and Health* (Boston & London: Shambhala, 1997).

Hewitt, J., *Meditation: Teach Yourself* (London: Hodder and Stoughton, 1989).

Ho, M.W., *The Rainbow and the Worm: The Physics of Organisms*, 2nd ed. (Singapore: World Scientific Publishing Company, 2003).

Jackson, M., *Pain: The Fifth Vital Sign: The Science and Culture of Why We Hurt* (New York: Crown Publishers, 2002).

Kabat-Zinn, J., *Full Catastrophe Living: How to Cope with Stress, Pain and Illness Using Mindfulness Meditation* (New York: Dell, 1990).

Kenyon, J., *21st Century Medicine* (London: Thorsons, 1986).

Khalsa, D.S., and C. Stauth, *Meditation as Medicine: Activate the Power of Your Natural Healing Force* (New York: Pocket Books, 2001).

Mason, K., *Thoughts that Harm, Thoughts that Heal: Overcoming Common Ailments Through the Power of Your Mind* (London: Piatkus, 2000).

Melzack, R., and P. Wall, *The Challenge of Pain* (London: Penguin Books, 1996).

Montagu, A., *Touching: The Human Significance of the Skin* (New York: Columbia University Press, 1971).

Sarno, J.E., *Mind over Back Pain* (New York: Berkeley Publishing Group, 1984).

Sarno, J.E., *Healing Back Pain* (New York: Warner Books, 1991).

Sarno, J.E., *The Mindbody Prescription* (New York: Warner Books, 1999).

Sears, B., *The Anti-Inflammation Zone* (New York: Regan Books, 2005).

Recommended Reading

Siler, B., *The Pilates Body* (London: Michael Joseph, 2000).

Sofaer, B., *Pain: Principles, Practice and Patients*, 3rd ed. (Cheltenham, U.K.: Stanley Thornes Publishing, 1998).

Wall, P., *The Science of Suffering* (London: Weidenfield and Nicolson, 1999).

Wells, P.E., V. Frampton, and D. Bowsher, *Pain Management by Physiotherapy*, 2nd ed. (Oxford, U.K.: Butterworth-Heinemann, 1997).

Williams, T., *The Complete Illustrated Guide to Chinese Medicine* (Shaftesbury Dorset, U.K.: Element Books, 1996).

Wittink, H., and M.T. Hoskins, eds., *Chronic Pain Management for Physiotherapists* (Newton, MA: Butterworth-Heinemann, 1997).

Worsley, J.R., *Acupuncture: Is It for You?* (Dorset Shaftesbury, U.K.: Element Books, 1990).

Resources

Author's Clinic

The Pain Management Practice
Our expert panel of consultants aims to provide pain relief and improved quality of life with physiotherapy, which includes electromedicine, acupuncture, and rehabilitation. We also include psychotherapy with relaxing breathwork exercises, emotional release in either group or individual sessions, and dietary advice to improve lifestyle and pain.

Phyllis Berger
E-mail: pberger@icon.co.za
Tel.: +27-11-883-2000
Fax: +27-11-883-3111
Website: www.easemypains.com

Organizations to Help with Pain

Some of the organizations listed below are geared to the layperson/pain sufferer, some to the practitioner. In addition to these websites, search on Google (or any other search engine) using keywords related to your condition, e.g., "chronic pain," "back pain," "CRPS," "fibromyalgia," etc.

American Pain Society *www.ampainsoc.org*

American Pain Foundation *www.painfoundation.org*

American Acupuncture Society *www.americanacupuncture.com*

Chronic Pain Support Group *www.chronicpainsupport.org*

Yahoo Member Groups (chat groups exist on the topics of chronic pain, CRPS, fibromyalgia, and many other conditions) *groups.yahoo.com*

British Pain Society *www.britishpainsociety.org*

British Medical Acupuncture Society *www.medical-acupuncture.co.uk*

Australian Pain Society *www.apsoc.org.au*

International Association for the Study of Pain (IASP) *www.iasp-pain.org*

European Federation of IASP Chapters *www.efic.org*

World Institute of Pain *www.worldinstituteofpain.org*

World Society of Pain Clinicians *www.painclinicians.org*

Equipment to Help with Pain

Acutouch *www.acutouch.com*

Alpha-Stim *www.alpha-stim.com*

Dynatron STS *www.dynatronics.com*

Magnets *www.magnetictherapysales.com* (in the U.K.: *www.magnetictherapy.co.uk*)

Other electrotherapy devices, TENS units, magnets, etc. *www.healiohealth.com*

TENS units *www.itolator.co.jp/English/profile.html*

APS Device (for administering modified direct current) *www.apstherapy.com*

APS Technologies is located in Hermanus, South Africa (e-mail: info@apstherapy.com). They are currently working with a U.S. distributor (DairyCell, based in North Bergen, NJ) to make the product available in North America. Until then, contact them directly via e-mail or website.

NMES (Winks Green Machine)

The device has been sold in many countries and is marketed in the United States by

Bulwark Electronics
P.O. Box 23891
Chattanooga TN 37422
(423) 899-2900
Fax: (423) 894-6611
(no website)

Index

A

A-beta fibers, 59, 66, 76, 79, 89
A-delta fibers, 59, 66, 76, 79, 89
abdominal muscles, 129–131
acetylcholine, 67
Achilles tendonitis, 212
action potential simulation current device (APS), *xxv*, 38, 89–93, and mood changes, 92; research on, 90–92; and sleep improvement, 92; and treatment of burns, 92. *See also* modified direct current (MDC)
acupoints, 65, 66, 79
acupuncture, *xiii*, *xxiii*, 64–74, 101, 102; acupoints, 65, 66; effectiveness of, 66–69; electroacupuncture, 69; and the emotions, 70–71; instructions for treatment, 157–158; integrative neuromuscular acupoint system, 177; intramuscular stimulation (IMS), 179–180; meridians, 65; and movement, 70; periosteal pecking, 61, 169, 177–178; plum-blossom needling, 61, 169, 178–179; for relaxation, 107; for stress reduction, 71–72; studies on, 69; subcutaneous needling, 179; techniques for ankle sprain, 164–165; techniques for back pain, 165–166; techniques for deafferentation (burning pain), 175–176; techniques for headaches, 169–171; techniques for inflammation, 160–161; techniques for knee pain, 166–169; techniques for neuralgia, 172; techniques for stress, 158–160; techniques for sympathetically mediated pain, 173–175; techniques for tendinomuscular meridian pain, 176; techniques for the autonomic nervous system, 162–164; techniques for the immune system, 161–162; techniques for wound/scar pain, 172; used with MDC therapy, 94
acupuncturist, 116
acute spasmodic nerve pain, 13
acutouch, 46–48, 147–148
adenosine, 90
adenosine triphosphate (ATP), 77, 89
adrenaline, 7, 8, 20, 60
afferent fibers, 59
AIDS, 108
Alexander technique, 97
allodynia, 2
allostasis, 4–5
Alpha-Stim, 86, 87
analgesia, temporary, 3
anesthetist, 116
anger, role of in pain, 7–8, 70
ankle sprain, acupuncture techniques for, 164–165
ankylosing spondylitis, 88, 90, 94, 120
anterior knee pain, 13–14
anti-inflammatory creams, 148
anticonvulsants, 7
antidepressants, 7
anxiety, 154
APS therapy. *See* action potential simulation current device
arachnoiditis, 175
aromatherapy, 148
arteriovenous malformation, 175
arthritis, 12, 46, 87, 90, 94, 102, 106, 148
arthropathies, 94
arthroscopy, 102, 111
ascending pathways, 61